AF615552

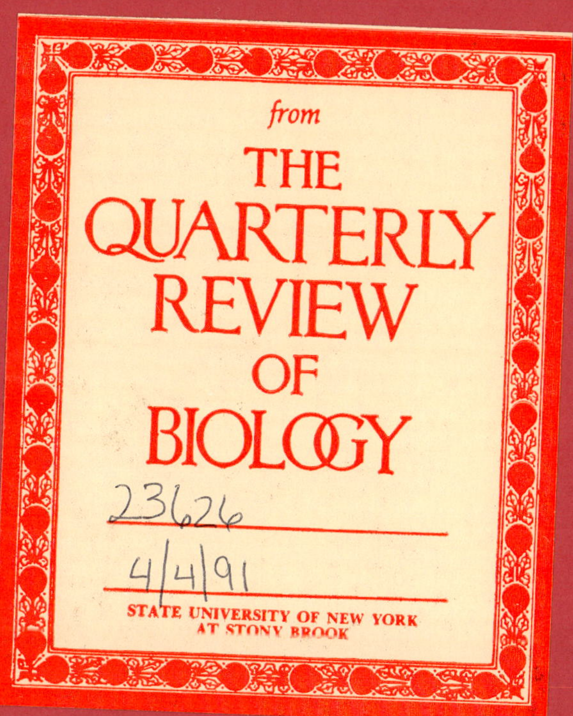
from
THE
QUARTERLY
REVIEW
OF
BIOLOGY
23626
4/4/91
STATE UNIVERSITY OF NEW YORK
AT STONY BROOK

Usibus Educto Si quicquam Credis Amicu.

—Cotton Mather, *The Angel of Bethesda*

Dictionary of Protopharmacology

Therapeutic Practices, 1700–1850

J. Worth Estes

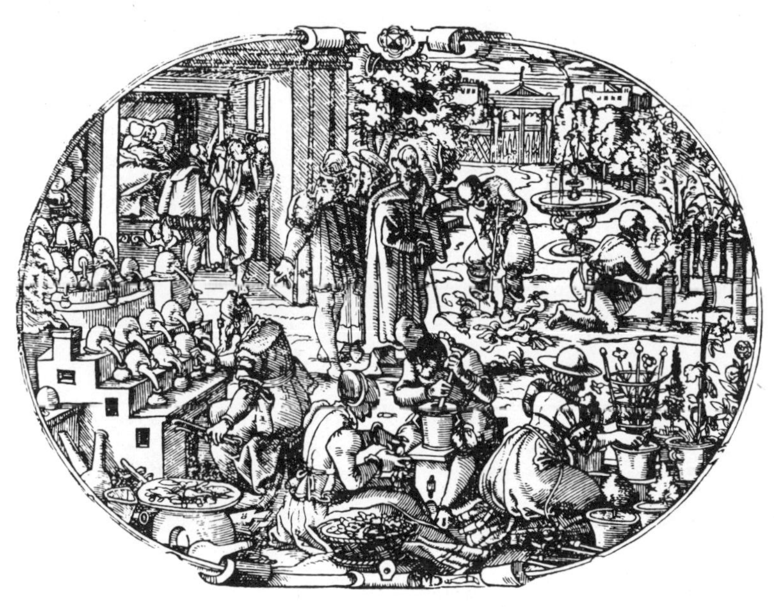

Science History Publications, U.S.A.
1990

First published in the United States of America
by Science History Publications/USA
a division of
Watson Publishing International
Post Office Box 493, Canton, MA 02021

Library of Congress Cataloging-in-Publication Data

Estes, J. Worth, 1934–
Dictionary of protopharmacology : therapeutic practices, 1700–1850
/ J. Worth Estes.
p. cm.
Includes bibliographical references.
ISBN 0-88135-068-0
1. Pharmacology—History—Dictionaries. 2. Materia medica—
Dictionaries. I. Title.
[DNLM: 1. Dictionaries, Pharmaceutic. 2. Pharmacology, Clinical—
history—dictionaries. QV 13 E79d]
RM36.E88 1990
615′.1′09033—dc20
DNLM/DLC
for Library of Congress 90-8628
CIP

Designed and manufactured in the U.S.A.

CONTENTS

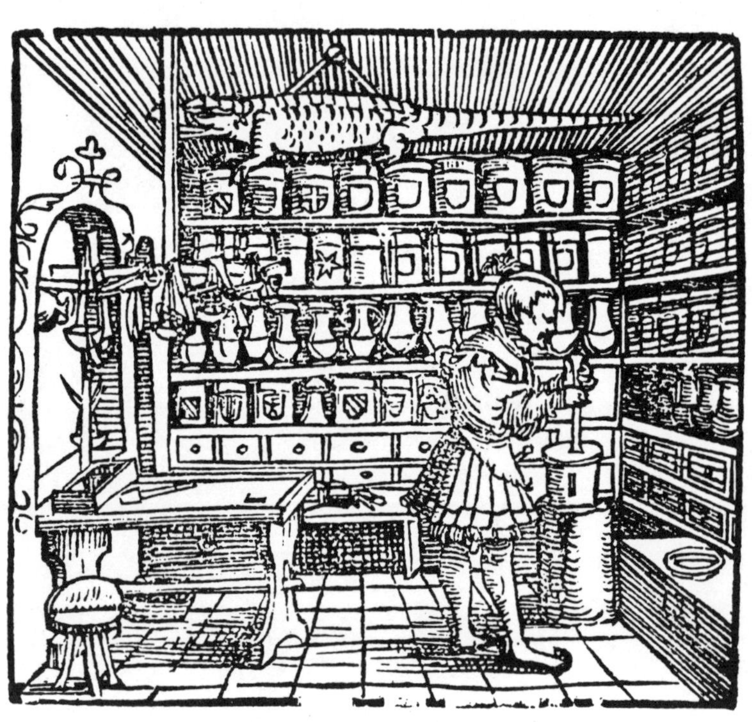

Directions for Use

As taught in modern medical schools, pharmacology is the study of drugs and their effects on living organisms. In 1975, Chauncey Leake, an eminent student of both modern and historical drugs, coined the word protopharmacology[1] to encompass the study of the drugs used during all the centuries before modern academic pharmacology began to emerge from the pioneering laboratory that Rudolph Bucheim established in Dorpat, Estonia, in 1849. Protopharmacological studies were almost exclusively empirical—that is, they were based chiefly on physicians' observations of their patients' responses to the drugs prescribed for them.

By contrast, Bucheim and his successors—led by Oswald Schmeideberg and, in the United States, John Jacob Abel—studied the sites and modes of drug action in intact animals and isolated tissues. Although similar methodologies had been used by investigators such as Claude Bernard and François Magendie as much as 20 years earlier, it was Bucheim's pupils whose work formed the nucleus of modern pharmacology, and their experimental approach is still integral to today's preclinical trials. Placebo-controlled clinical trials—which would have corrected many protopharmacological concepts—would not come into use until the 1940s.

The definitions collated in this dictionary have been designed to help students of historical medical practices identify the therapeutic terms that appear most often in English-language texts and manuscripts written during the century and a half before scientific laboratory studies began to dispel the medical profession's reliance on unproved—albeit time-tested—theories of how the body works in health and disease. Although the remedies defined here were selected for inclusion because they were used in general medical practice between about 1700 and 1850, many had entered medicine well before the time of Hippocrates, and many survived into the twentieth century. For instance, a large fraction of the drugs in this compendium—both botanical and chemical—can be found in the textbook of pharmacology used at the Harvard Medical School in 1909.[2] Although the dictionary emphasizes treatments employed by regular physicians, many of their drugs were also among those promoted by sectarian healers or by non-professionals, and for similar protopharmacological reasons. In addition, many purely "irregular" treatments and "patent" or proprietary medicines are included here. The list cannot encompass the entire range of historical drug usage, partly because the task might never end, and partly because the formulations of many preparations differed over time or from place to place.

I have focused most entries, and especially the cross-references, around the botanical nomenclatures and chemical concepts used in the 1794 edition of the *Edinburgh Dispensatory*, partly because its influence was pervasive on both sides of the Atlantic, and partly because it followed the major chemical discoveries of the eighteenth century. Dedicated to Joseph Black, M.D., professor of chemistry at Edinburgh, the dispensatory includes a helpful prefatory synopsis of Lavoisier's chemical discoveries. Similarly, items that first entered medical usage in the United States are cross-indexed to the nomenclature used in James Thacher's *American New Dispensatory* of 1813. All identifying chemical and botanical names given in the definitions are modern.

Scholars who need more detailed information about methods of drug preparation should consult pharmacopoeias appropriate to the time and place of their study for exact ingredients of specific drugs and methods of compounding them. Much of the information in this dictionary has been derived chiefly from dispensatories and textbooks because they were more concerned with drugs' clinical uses than were the pharmacopoeias. However, since pathophysiological concepts as well as the clinical indications for each drug or ingredient varied from time to time and from one physician to the next, only minimal attention is given here to the specific diagnoses, or *diseases*, for which each drug was used (or said to have been used). As Marie-François-Xavier Bichat (1771-1802) taught, "The same drugs were successively used by humoralists and solidists. Theories changed, but the drugs remained the same. They were applied and acted in the same way, which proves that their action is independent of the opinion of doctors."[3]

Therefore, I have listed the ways in which each item in the materia medica was thought to affect the body in terms of the sites and modes of drug action that were inherent in the definitions of the drug classes that physicians recognized in the eighteenth and nineteenth centuries (e.g., astringents, diaphoretics, emetics, narcotics, and so forth, terms that are also defined here). Thus, this dictionary provides a physician's-eye view of practical protopharmacology—although apothecaries and patients shared that view.

The enormous frequency with which drug properties such as diaphoretic, diuretic, and emetic are listed here underscores the observation that "the physician's most potent weapon was his ability to 'regulate the secretions.' "[4] Similarly, the frequency with which drug properties such as astringent, anti-inflammatory, antispasmodic, discutient, febrifuge, and resolvent occur alerts us to the eighteenth-century concept of fever as a "spasmodic affection." As the 1771 first edition of the *Encyclopaedia Britannica* pointed out in its entry on medicine, "Whatever has a power to irritate . . . the nervous and vascular system to spasms is most likely to generate a fever."[5]

Each protopharmacologic drug class could be—and was—applied to several different specific diseases now known to be unrelated. Furthermore, members of several different drug classes were often judged to be effective treatments for any one diagnosis. The physician's principal therapeutic goal was to modulate both the body's secretions and any pathogenic irritations of its vascular and nervous tissue fibers, regardless of what had disturbed their equilibria in the first place. I have used the present tense in defining the modes of action and side effects of most drugs, because the physicians who prescribed them would have used that tense in describing their remedies. Tacit evidence that these concepts have regularly frustrated historians, as Rosenberg has noted,[6] appears in the nearly total neglect of all but the most bizarre or the most "modern" therapies in standard histories of medicine, like those of Garrison, Shryock, and Major.

Many preparations with more than one active ingredient are included here; preparations with only one major ingredient are not given definitions other than those necessary to describe that ingredient (e.g., both tinctures and oxymels of any given material were usually understood to have the same kind of therapeutic effect), since the exact preparation prescribed was chosen chiefly to maximize the patient's exposure to the drug. Similarly, preparations with two or three ingredients, all of which were specified in the name of the preparation, are not defined separately unless the combination had one or more effects that could not have been predicted from their individual properties (e.g., Pulvis Aloes cum Canella).

The reference numbers given in square brackets [ ] are to items among the General References below that can be consulted for more details about the main entry's presumed role in clinical practice. Unless clearly specified at the end of an entry, no modern concepts of the drugs' pharmacological effects are given here. A few entries include additional references to helpful modern studies of their historical usage, their pharmacologic properties, or their toxicity.

Words capitalized within the definitions will be found as separate entries (as can the names of drug classes and properties given in lower case). Major entries begin with a modern identification, insofar as possible, of the drug or its ingredients. For a few inorganic compounds of uncertain identity, the method of preparation is given. Not all identifications of plant or animal species, or of inorganic chemicals, are as precise as some might have wished, especially in the wake of changing scientific nomenclatures. However, it seems unlikely that conclusions about their clinical applications or their therapeutic efficacy will be affected by such imprecision.

When possible, the circumstances under which each drug entered the materia medica are noted. This has been possible chiefly for those first discovered in the New World; most of the others had been used by Old World physicians since antiquity or were introduced, largely through alchemy, in the late middle ages and the early Reniassance. In addition, notes about the isolation of the pharmacologically active components of botanical remedies are appended when appropriate.

Eponymous compounds are alphabetized by the proper name. Users of this dictionary should be wary of alternative spellings; slight familiarity with the common declensions and verb forms of classical Latin will help solve many questions about both spelling and chemical nomenclature before it achieved its modern standardization.

Several non-drug therapeutic modes (e.g., bleeding, bougie, diet, electricity, and heat) are included, partly because they were applied clinically within the physiological concepts that were used to explain drug action, and partly to assist the research of scholars who are not yet familiar with such methods. However, other sources should be consulted for further details. Entries on dose and measurement explain the weights and measures used in compounding drugs, and list many common abbreviations for them. As is apparent in several entries, eighteenth-century physicians were well aware of the dose-effect relationship that has been the keystone of modern pharmacological studies since the 1920s.

The following generic terms, most of which reflect compounding procedures, are not used in alphabetization (e.g., Aqua Calcis is found as Calcis, Aqua):

ACETUM
AETHER (or ETHER)
AQUA
BACCAE (berries)
BALSAM[UM]
CATAPLASM
CORTEX (bark)
CRYSTALLI
DECOCTUM (or DECOCTION)
ELIXIR
EMULSIO[N]
EMPLASTRUM (or PLASTER)
EXTRACT[UM]
FLOWERS (or FLORES)
FOLIA (leaves)
GUM
INFUSUM (or INFUSION)
LAC (or MILK)
LINIMENTUM
LIQUOR
MEL (honey)
MISTURA (or MIXTURA)
OINTMENT
OL or OLEUM (oil)
OXYMEL
PILL (or PILULE)
POTERUS or POTUS (drink)
POWDER (or PULVIS)
RADIX (root)
SAL[T]
SEMINA (seeds)
SOLUTIO[N]
SPIRITUS (or SPIRITS)
SUCCUS (juice)
SYRUP[US]
TINCTURA (or TINCTURE)
UNGUENTUM
VINUM

NOTES

1. Chauncey D. Leake, *An Historical Account of Pharmacology to the Twentieth Century* (Springfield, Ill.: Charles C. Thomas, 1975), p. 17.
2. Maurice Vejux Tyrode, *Pharmacology: the Actions and Uses of Drugs* (Philadephia: P. Blakiston's Son & Co., 1908). Harvard was not uniquely anachronistic in this respect; several agents that appear in this dictionary can still be found in current textbooks.
3. Quoted in Erwin H. Ackerknecht, *Medicine at the Paris Hospital*, 1794-1848 (Baltimore: Johns Hopkins Press, 1967), p. 131.
4. Charles E. Rosenberg, "The Therapeutic Revolution: Medicine, Meaning, and Social Change in Nineteenth-Century America," *Perspectives in Biology and Medicine 20* (1977): 485-506.
5. *Encyclopaedia Britannica*, 3 vols. (Edinburgh: A. Bell and C. Macfarquhar, 1771), III, pp. 486-487.
6. Rosenberg, "Therapeutic Revolution," n. 4.

ILLUSTRATIONS

The botanical headpieces and tailpieces that accompany the letters of the alphabet are from Nicholas Lémery's *Dictionnaire Universel des Drogues Simples* (Paris: L.-Ch. d'Houry, 1759). The cut on the title page is from the title page of Jacobus Theodorus' *Ein new Artzney Buch* (Newstadt an der Hardt: Mattheum Harnisch, 1592). The cut of the apothecary in his shop is from Walther Hermann Ryff's *ConfectBuch und Hauss-Apoteck. Kuenstlich zubereiten, einmachen, und gebrauchen, wes in ordenlichen Apotecker* (Franckfurt: Bei Chr. Egen. Erben., 1563). All of the illustrations are reproduced by courtesy of the Boston Medical Library.

GENERAL REFERENCES

1. J. Worth Estes, "Drug Usage at the Infirmary: the Example of Dr. Andrew Duncan, Sr.," Appendix D to: Guenter B. Risse, *Hospital Life in Enlightenment Scotland: Care and Teaching at the Royal Infirmary of Edinburgh* (New York: Cambridge University Press, 1986), pp. 351-384. (The detailed clinical cases in Appendix B also provide unusual insights into late 18th-century therapeutic thinking.)

2. J. Worth Estes, "Therapeutic Practice in Colonial New England," in Philip Cash, Eric H. Christianson, and J. Worth Estes, eds., *Medicine in Colonial Massachusetts, 1620-1820* (Boston: Colonial Society of Massachusetts, 1980), pp. 289-383.

3. J. Worth Estes, "John Jones' *Mysteries of Opium Reveal'd* (1701): Key to Historical Opiates," *Journal of the History of Medicine and Allied Sciences 34* (1979): 200-209.

4. J. Worth Estes, *Hall Jackson and The Purple Foxglove: Medical Practice and Research in Revolutionary America, 1760-1820* (Hanover, N.H.: University Press of New England, 1979).

5. J. Worth Estes, "Naval Medicine in the Age of Sail: the Voyage of the *New York*, 1802-1803," *Bulletin of the History of Medicine 56* (1982): 238-253.

6. J. Worth Estes and LaVerne Kuhnke, "French Observations of Disease and Drug Use in Late Eighteenth-Century Cairo," *Journal of the History of Medicine and Allied Sciences 39* (1984): 121-152.

7. J. Worth Estes, "The Pharmacology of Nineteenth-Century Patent Medicines," *Pharmacy in History 30* (1988): 3-18.

8. J. Worth Estes, *The Medical Skills of Ancient Egypt* (Canton, Mass.: Science History Publications, 1989).

9. J. Worth Estes, "Making Therapeutic Decisions with Protopharmacologic Evidence," *Transactions and Studies of the College of Physicians of Philadelphia n.s. 1* (1979): 116-137.

10. Thomas Palmer, *The Admirable Secrets of Physick and Chyrurgery*, Thomas Rogers Forbes, ed. (New Haven, Yale University Press, 1984).

11. John Millar, *Observations on the Prevailing Diseases in Great Britain* (London: for the author, 1798).

12. *The Practice of the British and French Hospitals*, 2nd ed. (London: R. Baldwin, 1775).

13. A. C. Wootton, *Chronicles of Pharmacy*, 2 vols. in 1 (1910; rprt. ed. Boston: Milford House, 1971).

14. George B. Griffenhagen and James Harvey Young, *Old*

English Patent Medicines in America. Contributions from the Museum of History and Technology, United States National Museum Bulletin 218 (Washington, DC: Smithsonian Institution, 1959), pp. 155-183.
15. *Edinburgh New Dispensatory*, 4th ed. (Edinburgh: William Creech, G.G. Robinson, and T, Kay, 1794).
16. Leslie G. Matthews, "Daybook of the Court Apothecary in the Time of William and Mary, 1691," *Medical History 22* (1978): 161-173.
17. P. S. Brown, "Medicines Advertised in Eighteenth-Century Bath Newspapers," *Medical History 20* (1976): 152-168.
18. S. J., "Drugs Used at Hudson Bay in 1730," *Bulletin of the New York Academy of Medicine 47* (1971): 838-842.
19. Nicholas Lémery, *Pharmacopée Universelle*, ed. 5 (Paris, 1763).
20. John Huxham, *An Essay on Fevers* (1757; rprt. ed., Canton, Mass.: Science History Publications, 1986).
21. Kenneth F. Lampe and Mary Ann McCann, *AMA Handbook of Poisonous and Injurious Plants* (Chicago: American Medical Association, 1985).
22. Robert Thomas, *Modern Domestic Medicine* (New York: Collins and Co., 1829).
23. James Thacher, *The American New Dispensatory*, 2nd ed. (Boston: Thomas B. Wait and Co. and C. Williams, 1813).
24. Faculté de Médecine de Paris, *Codex Medicamentarius* (Paris: Guillelmus Cavelier, 1748).
25. Moyse Charas, *Pharmacopée Royale Galenique et Chymique* (Lyon: Freres Bruyset, 1753).
26. M. J. Cartheuser, *Matière Médicale*, 4 vols. (Paris: Briasson, 1755).
27. Friedrich A. Flückiger and Daniel Hanbury, *Pharmacographia: A History of the Principal Drugs of Vegetable Origin* (London: Macmillan and Co., 1874). (Invaluable for historical details and bibliographies.)
28. Roger Tory Peterson and Margaret McKenny, *A Field Guide to Wildflowers* (Boston: Houghton Mifflin, 1968).
29. George B. Wood and Franklin Bache, *The Dispensatory of the United States of America*, 8th ed. (Philadelphia: Grigg, Elliott, and Co., 1849).
30. Jacob Bigelow, *A Treatise on the Materia Medica* (Boston: Charles Ewer, 1822).
31. Eric W. Martin, ed., *Remington's Pharmaceutical Sciences*, 13th ed. (Easton, Penna: Mack Publishing Co., 1965).

32. Robert Thomas, *Modern Domestic Medicine* (New York: Collins and Co., 1829).
33. Louis Goodman and Alfred Gilman, *The Pharmacological Basis of Therapeutics* (New York, Macmillan Co., 1940; 2nd ed., 1955; 3rd ed., 1965; 4th ed., 1970; 5th ed., 1975; 6th ed., 1980; 7th ed., 1985).
34. Harold William Rickett, *Wild Flowers of the United States. Volume One: The Northeastern States*, 2 parts (New York: New York Botanical Garden & McGraw-Hill Book Co., 1966).
35. R[obert] James, *A Medicinal Dictionary*, 3 vols. (London: T. Osborne, 1743-1745). (This monumental work contains detailed formulas for hundreds of compounded remedies that are not included in the present work because by 1700 they were already of more historical than therapeutic importance. Nevertheless, these volumes will be of great value in deciphering drug names given in materials written before the 18th century.)
36. Ann Leighton, *Early American Gardens: "For Meate or Medicine"* (Boston: Houghton Mifflin Co., 1970). (Contains a useful appendix on uses of botanical remedies in the 17th-century home.)
37. Ann Leighton, *American Gardens in the Eighteenth Century: "For Use or for Delight"* (Boston: Houghton Mifflin Co., 1976).
38. Ann Leighton, American Gardens of the Nineteenth Century: "For Comfort and Affluence" (Amherst, Mass.: University of Massachusetts Press, 1987).
39. Saul Jarcho, *The Clinical Consultations of Giambattista Morgagni* (Boston: Countway Library of Medicine and Science History Publications, 1984). (This and the next reference provide the best windows into early 18th-century therapeutic reasoning available in print.)
40. Saul Jarcho, *Clinical Consultations and Letters by Ippolito Francesco Albertini, Francesco Torti, and Other Physicians* (Boston: Countway Library of Medicine and Science History Publications, 1989).
41. Fielding H. Garrison, *An Introduction to the History of Medicine*, 4th ed. (Philadelphia: W. B. Saunders Co., 1929).
42. B. Holmstedt and G. Liljestrand, *Readings in Pharmacology* (New York: Macmillan Co., 1963).
43. Thomas E. Keys, *The History of Surgical Anesthesia* (1945; rprt. ed., Huntington, N.Y.: Robert E. Krieger Publishing Co., 1978).
44. Paul G. Stecher, ed. *The Merck Index*, 7th ed. (Rahway, N.J.: Merck & Co., 1960).

45. T. E. Wallis, *Textbook of Pharmacognosy*, 4th ed. (London, J. & A. Churchill, Ltd., 1960).
46. J. Worth Estes, "Quantitative Observations of Fever and its Treatment before the Advent of Short Clinical Thermometers," *Medical History* (in press for 1991).

ACKNOWLEDGEMENTS

Over the years, many historical drugs have been brought to my attention by friends and colleagues simply because they thought I would like to know about them, because I had asked about them, or while we were collaborating on a project of mutual interest. Those who have contributed in one of more of those ways include Rosemary Angel (Kew Gardens, London), Dr. Paul Berman (Amherst, Mass.), Dr. Harold J. Cook (Madison, Wisc.), David L. Cowen (Jamesburg, N.J.), Ira Dye (Virginia Beach, Va.), Josephine Gladstone (Hawarden, Clwyd, Wales), David Gunner (Harvard Medical School), Ida Hay (Arnold Arboretum, Boston), Dr. Gregory J. Higby (Institute for the History of Pharmacy, Madison, Wisc.), Dr. LaVerne Kuhnke (Northeastern University, Boston), Dr. Marjorie Lemay (Boston), Dr. Adam G. N. Moore (Boston), Dr. Edward W. Pelikan (Boston University), Dr. Guenter B. Risse (University of California, San Francisco), and Dr. Fatima M. Sa'ad (Dokki Agricultural Station, Cairo, Egypt), among others; to all of them my warmest thanks. I am also grateful to Professor Cowen for his expert and gracious comments on an early draft of the manuscript. And I owe a great debt to Joyce Becotte, who patiently word-processed my endless corrections and humored all my changing ideas on the format of the manuscript.

Richard J. Wolfe, Curator of Rare Books and Manuscripts at the Francis A. Countway Library of Medicine in Boton, and Garland Librarian of the Boston Medical Library, has earned my deepest appreciation for his major contributions to my thinking about historical drugs, especially because he has unerringly steered me to the best available reflections of drug usage in the past. This book is for him.

J.W.E.

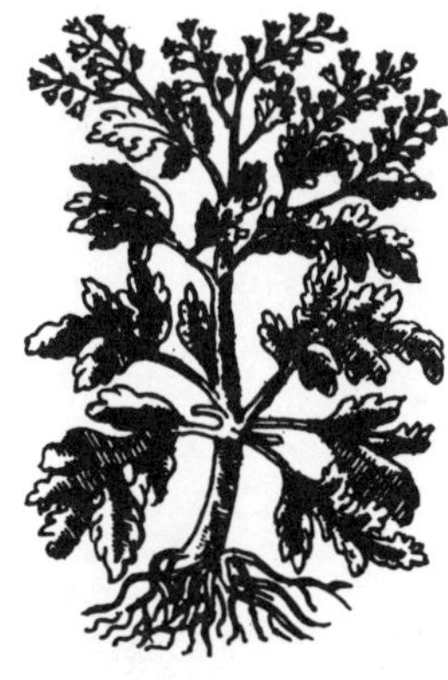

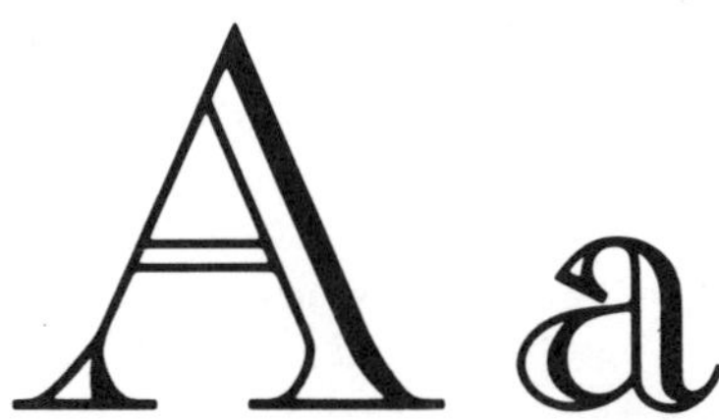

Artemisia

aa: Abbreviation for *ana*, "of each," used in prescription writing.

ABBE BLONDEL'S CHYMICAL SPECIFICK: A proprietary prophylaxis and remedy for venereal disease.

ABELMOSCHUS: Seeds of "musk," *Hibiscus esculentus*. Aromatic. [15]

ABIES: Same as BALSAMUM CANADENSE.

ABIETIS, ACIDUM: Water extract of resins from *Pinus abies* or *P. sylvestris*. Diaphoretic, diuretic, and antiscorbutic. Also see TEREBINTHA entries. [15]

ABIETIS, BALSAM: Same as BALSAMUM CANADENSE.

ABROTANUM: Extract of southernwood, *Artemisia abrotanum*. Anthelminthic, tonic, and diaphoretic; applied externally as a discutient, antiseptic, and to prevent hair loss. [15]

ABSINTHUM (or ABSINTHIUM) [VULGARE]: Leaves and flowering tops of common wormwood, *Artemisia absinthum*. A strong bitter and stimulant tonic with an offensive taste; antispasmodic, stomachic, diuretic, febrifuge, narcotic, and emmenagogue; the oil can also be used as a vermifuge, and the leaves applied externally as an antiseptic and discutient. Wine of absinthe was invented by Dr. Ordinaire and its recipe was sold to Pernod in 1797. [15,23,29] See: Wilfred Niels Arnold, "Absinthe," *Scientific American*, June, 1989, pp. 112-117, and his "Vincent Van Gogh and the Thujone Connection," *Journal of the American Medical Association 260* (1988): 3042-3044; and Donald G. Vogt, "Absinthium: a Nineteenth Century Drug of Abuse," *Journal of Ethnopharmacology 4* (1981): 337-342. Thujone, the intoxicating convulsant ingredient of absinthe, was isolated by Leblanc in 1845.

ABSINTHUM MARITIMUM: Small top leaves of sea wormwood, *Artemisia maritima*. Diuretic and corroborant. [15]

ABSINTHUM, SAL: Same as LIXIVA.

Absorbent: An alkaline agent that absorbs noxious materials from the body. By the 1790s, most absorbents were being reclassified as antacids.

Abstergent: Essentially, a detergent.

ACACIAE GUMMI: Same as GUM ARABIC.

ACACIA GERMANICA: Same as PRUNUS SYLVESTRIS.

ACACIA VERA: Juice of unripe fruit of *Acacia senegal* (formerly *Mimosa nilotica*); also see GUM ARABIC. Mild astringent. [15]

ACETIS HYDRARGYRI: Mercurous acetate. Undependable antisyphilitic; see HYDRARGYRUS. [23]

ACETIS PLUMBI: Same as CERUSSA ACETATA.

ACETIS POTASSAE: Potassium acetate; see DIURETIC SALT.

ACETITIS AMMONIAE, AQUA: Same as AQUA AMMONIAE ACETATAE.

ACETITIS PLUMBI ET IPECACUANHAE, PILULE: Pill made with CERUSSA ACETATA, IPECAC, and OPIUM. Astringent, for internal and uterine bleeding. [23]

ACETITIS ZINCI, SOLUTIO: Solution of zinc acetate, for intraurethral injection for gonorrhea (i.e., spermatorrhea). [23]

ACETOSA: Extract of leaves of sour-grass, or wood-sorrel, *Rumex acetellosa*. Refrigerant, diuretic, aperient, and antiscorbutic; roots regarded as deobstruent and diuretic, and the seeds as antidiarrheal. [15,23,29] Also see LUJULA, and RUMEX entries.

ACETOSELLAE, SAL: Oxalic acid (actually, a mixture of potassium binoxalate and tetroxalate); see RUMEX entries.

ACETOSUM, ACIDUM: Acetic acid, found in vinegar; sometimes used to mean vinegar (see ACETUM). Tonic and rubefacient. [23]

Acetum: A vinegar solution of a drug, sometimes with PROOF SPIRIT added.

ACETUM: Vinegar. Mild diuretic and refrigerant, often used when an acid is indicated. [15] Strong antiseptic; astringent tonic; sometimes used in glysters, liniments, and gargles. [23,29,30]

ACETUM AROMATICUM: A mixture of ROSMARINUS, SALVIA, LAVENDULA, and CARYOPHYLLUS, in ACETUM. Used as an antiseptic fumigant in sick chambers. [15] Also see VINAIGRE DES QUATRE VOLEURS.

ACETUM OPII: Fermented vinegar of OPIUM, but of unpredictable efficacy. [30]

ACETUM VINI: Wine vinegar, produced by a second fermentation of wines. Administered internally and externally for its anti-inflammatory and antiseptic properties; also used in extracting the active principles of botanical drugs. [15]

ACID DROPS: Probably ELIXIR VITRIOL.

ACIDI CARBONIC, AQUA: Carbonic acid water, or artificial SODA WATER.

ACIDUS, SYRUPUS: Mixture of VITRIOLICUM DILUTUM and syrup of LIMON. Astringent. [15]

ACIPENSER STURIO: Same as ICHTHYOCOLLA.

ACONITUM: Leaves of wolfsbane (or monk's hood), *Aconitum napellum*. Vigorously promoted by Dr. Anton Störck of Vienna in 1762 for use in a wide range of illnesses characterized by swollen glands or painful joints. Narcotic, tonic, diaphoretic, and diuretic. [23,29] Its side effects include vomiting, diarrhea, bradycardia, bradypnea, vertigo, delirium, convulsions, coma, and death. [15,23] The plant's active alkaloid, aconitine, isolated by Philipp Lorenz Geiger and Germain Henri Hess of Heidelberg in 1833, produces dysarthria, distorted vision, vomiting, and cardiac arrhythmias.

ACORUS: See CALAMUS AROMATICUS.

ACTEA SPICATA: Root of herb christopher, or red baneberry, *Actaea rubra*. Astringent tonic. Poisonous. [23]

ADDER'S-TONGUE: See ERYTHRONIUM.

ADEPS: Same as AXUNGUENTUM PORCINUM.

ADIPIS SUILLAE: Lard mixed with mutton suet.

AERATA, AQUA (or AQUA AERIS FIXI): "Aerial," or carbonic, acid, prepared by dissolving chalk (calcium carbonate) in sulfuric acid and then saturating spring water with the evolving gas, which was FIXED AIR (carbon dioxide). [1,15]

AERUGINIS AMMONIATAE, AQUA: "Ammoniated copper," VERDEGRIS in AQUA AMMONIAE. Used externally for skin ulcers, and, after dilution, as a collyrium. [15]

AERUGINIS, OXYMEL: "Oxymel of copper," VERDEGRIS in honey and vinegar. Used for cleaning skin sores, and for venereal sores in the mouth. [15]

AERUGINIS, UNGUENTUM: "Ointment of VERDEGRIS." Used to clean skin sores, because of copper's tonic property, and as a collyrium for ophthalmia. [15]

AERUGO: Same as VERDEGRIS.

AESCULUS: See HIPPOCASTANUM.

Aether: A very volatile spirit.

Aethiops: A dark or black substance.

AETHIOPS FERRI, or AETHIOPS IRON: Ferrous oxide.

AETHIOPS MARTIALIS: FERRI RUBIGO in OL OLIVA. Tonic.

AETHIOPS MEDICINALIS [PLUMMER'S]: Same as PLUMMER'S POWDER.

AETHIOPS MINERALIS: Same as HYDRARGYRUS SULPHURATUS NIGER.

AETHIOPS NARCOTICUS: HYDRARGYRUS dissolved in nitric acid and precipitated with KALI SULPHURATUM. Introduced from Germany to Britain in late 18th century for its narcotic effect (which was ascribed to its sulfur content). Side effects include confusion and vertigo. Because it "keeps the belly open," said to be superior to OPIUM, which regularly produces constipation. [1]

AETHIOPS VEGETABILIS: Mixture of OPIUM and VINUM. Suppresses hemorrhage and other discharges (e.g., diarrhea).

AGARICUS: A fungus, *Boletus igniarius* (so-called because it is easily flammable), used as a styptic. [15]

AGRIMONIA: Leaves of agrimony, *Agrimonia eupatoria*. Aperient, detergent, and tonic. [15]

AGRIMONY, HEMP: See EUPATORIUM.

AGRIPPAE, UNGUENTUM: Same as UNGUENTUM DIABRYONIAS; said to have been invented by one of the two kings of Jerusalem named Agrippa, but perhaps by

16th–century German physician Cornelius Heinrich Agrippa (von Nettesheim).

AJUGA: See CHAMAEPITHYS.

ALBA, UNGUENT: "White ointment," made of OL OLIVA, CERA ALBA, and LITHARGE. A plaster for burns. [2]

ALBUM RHASIS: "White [lead] of Rhazes," the famous late 9th-century Persian physician; same as UNGUENTUM CERUSSA ACETATAE.

ALCHEMILLA: Leaves of ladies' mantle, *Alchemilla vulgaris* (but possibly a *Spiranthes* spp.). Uterine tonic; antidiarrheal. [15]

ALCOHOL (or ALKOHOL): Distilled from SPIRITUS VINOSUS RECTIFICATUS over KALI or some other alkaline salt, to retain the water in the heated vessel, until the specific gravity fell from 0.8333-0.835 to 0.815. To make 100 proof alcohol, 20 oz. of alcohol were added to 17 oz. of distilled water. Tonic, carminative, and digestive; used in liniments to stimulate local blood flow. [23,29] The pioneering account of alcoholism was published by Dr. John Coakley Lettsom in 1789. Also see VINUM.

ALCOHOL AMMONIATUM: Same as SPIRITUS AMMONIAE.

ALCORNOQUE, [DIVINE]: Wood of one of the cork-oaks, *Byrsonima* spp. Tonic, astringent; reported, in 1810, to be a remedy for tuberculosis and liver disease. [23, pp. 370-373]

ALDER: See ALNUS and PRINOS.

ALEMBROTH, SAL: A mixture of SAL AMMONIAC and CALOMEL.

ALE[O]PHANGINAE, PILULE: An aromatic cathartic of which the chief ingredient was ALOES.

ALETRIS: Root of colic-root, or stargrass, *Aletris farinosa*. Tonic and stomachic; produces nausea, catharsis, and emesis as dose increases; also, narcotic. [29,30]

ALEXANDRINA, AUREA: See AUREA ALEXANDRINA.

Alexipharmic: Originally, an antidote against poison, but by the late 18th century it meant a medicine with antiseptic and diaphoretic properties. It was also often a synonym for HUXHAM'S TINCTURE. One formulation was said to be "an excellent medicine in contagious fevers, especially when the pulse and spirits are low and languid." [12] Also see Alexiteric.

Alexiteric: An antidote against poison; originally, a remedy for the bite of a venomous animal. Also see Alexipharmic.

ALGAROTH'S POWDER: Same as MERCURIUS VITAE.

ALHANDAL: Same as COLOCYNTHIS.

ALKALI FIXUM VEGETABILE: Potassium hydroxide.

ALKALINA AERATA, AQUA: Aerated alkaline solution prepared by saturating 2 oz. of LIXIVA dissolved in one gal. water with FIXED AIR. [1]

ALKALINE LIXIVA, CAUSTIC: Same as LYE.

ALKALINE SALT: Sodium carbonate. Lithontriptic. [2]

ALKALINUS FIXUS FOSSILIS, SAL: Same as BARILLA.

ALKALINUS FIXUS VEGETABILIS, SAL: Potassium hydroxide.

ALKALINUS, SYRUPUS: Mixture of SAL TARTARI and simple syrup. Antacid. [15]

Alkaloid: Literally, "alkali–like." The word was coined in 1818 by K. F. W. Meissner of Halle, to identify weak bases derived from plants. Now applied to nitrogen–containing materials found in plants.

ALKANET: Henna, the red dye extracted from the leaves and shoots of the North African species *Lawsonia inermis* or *L. alba*. For coloring only.

ALKEKENGI: Fruits of winter cherries, or jack-o'lanterns, *Physalis alkekengi*. Aperient; diuretic. [15]

ALKERMES: Same as KERMES.

ALLIARIA: Leaves of sauce-alone, *Erysimum alliaria*. Internally, diaphoretic and deobstruent; externally, antiseptic. [15]

ALLIUM: Usually, GARLIC; however, in a few cases, onion, or CEPA, may have been meant. [1]

ALLSPICE: See PIMENTO.

ALMONDS: See AMYGDALA.

ALNUS: Leaves and bark of alder, *Alnus* spp. Styptic. [15]

ALOE[S]: Inspissated juice of *Aloe perfoliata* or *A. barbadensis*; the best grade, known as Socotrine (or Socotorine), was said to come from Socotrina Island in the Arabian Sea; a slightly lesser grade was called Hepatica, while the crudest was Caballine or Horse (i.e., "coarse") aloes. Most often used as a warm stimulating cathartic that operates slowly but reliably, sometimes producing bloody stools; also, anthelminthic and emmenagogue. [1,15,23,29] Still used as a cathartic, by virtue of its ability to irritate the colon.

ALOES COMPOSITA, TINCTURA: Alcohol extract of ALOES, CROCUS, and MYRRH. Warm stimulant, stomachic, aperient, cathartic; diaphoretic, diuretic; antihysteric, emmenagogue. Sometimes made with added AETHER VITRIOLICUS, for patients with hot constitutions and weak stomachs. Occasionally used as a surgical dressing. [2,15]

ALOES CUM COLOCYNTHIDE, PILULE: Pill made with ALOES, SCAMMONY, VITRIOL ANTIMONIUM, COLOCYNTHIS, CARYOPHYLLUS AROMATICUS, and GUM ARABIC. Cathartic; cephalic. [1,15] Also see COCCIA.

ALOES CUM GUAIACUM, PILULE or PULVIS: Pill or powder of ALOES and GUAIAC. In small doses, diaphoretic; cathartic in large doses. [15]

ALOES PILL (or ALOETICAE, PILULE): Made with ALOES, GENTIAN, and simple syrup. [1,15]

ALOES, TINCTURA: Alcohol extract of Socotrine ALOES and GLYCERRHIZA. Cathartic. [15]

ALOES (or ALOETICUM), VINUM: Mixture of Socotrine ALOES, CANELLA, CARDAMOMUM MINUS, and ZINGIBER in Spanish white wine (sometimes with PROOF SPIRIT added). Cathartic, tonic. [15]

Alterative: A medicine that corrects or evacuates foul humors by unexplained mechanisms; may also affect the peripheral circulation (as manifested by an altered pulse rate).

ALTHAEA [OFFICINALIS]: Gummy extract of roots of *Althaea officinalis*, marsh mallow. Used as a non-specific binding agent; as an emollient and demulcent, especially in cataplasms; and in drinks for patients with renal colic, and in enemas. [1]

ALTHAEA, FERNEL'S SYRUP OF: A general deobstruent made with ALTHAEA and many other ingredients that was devised in 1593 (probably not invented by Dr. Jean Fernel of Paris, who died in 1558).

ALUM[EN]: Alum, potassium aluminum sulfate. A potent astringent and antispasmodic for internal and topical use. Side effects: nausea, vomiting, catharsis, and constipation. [1,23,29]

ALUMINIS COMPOSITA, AQUA: "Compound water of alum." Aqueous solution of ALUM and ZINCUM VITRIOLATUM. Used for cleaning skin ulcers and wounds, and cutaneous eruptions; as a collyrium; and for intraurethral injection for gonorrhea (i.e., spermatorrhea), or intravaginal administration for leukorrhea. [15]

ALUMINIS COMPOSITA, PULVIS: "Compound powder of alum." Styptic powder derived from PULVIS STYPTICUS HELVETII, made with ALUM and GUM KINO. [15]

ALUMINOSAE, AQUAE: "Aluminated waters." Medicinal waters closely resembling MAGNESIA VITRIOLATA.

ALUM ROOT: See HEUCHERA.

AMARA, TINCTURA: "Bitter tincture," a stomachic elixir; usually same as VINUM AMARUM. [2]

AMARUM, INFUSUM: "Bitter infusion," a water extract of GENTIAN, CORTEX AURANTIUM, CORIANDRUM, and PROOF SPIRIT. Carminative, stomachic, and a general tonic for the vascular system. [1]

AMARUM, VINUM: "Bitter wine," a mixture of GENTIAN, CINCHONA, CORTEX AURANTIUM, and CANELLA in PROOF SPIRIT and/or Spanish white wine. Stomachic. [15]

AMBER: See SUCCINUM.

AMBRAGRISEA: Ambergris; thought to be same as SPERMACETI, but formed in the intestines of the sperm whale and found floating in the sea.

AMMONIAC [or AMMONIACUM]: Almost always same as GUM AMMONIAC.

AMMONIACAL COPPER: Same as CUPRUM AMMONIACUM.

AMMONIAC, GUM: *Dorema ammoniacum* extract. A general stimulant, with antispasmodic, deobstruent, antihysteric, emmenagogue, expectorant, cathartic, diaphoretic, and diuretic properties; externally, an emollient and discutient. [2,15,23,29]

AMMONIACI, LAC: "Milk of ammonia," GUM AMMONIAC emulsified in water. Expectorant. [2]

AMMONIAC[US], SAL: Ammonium chloride. Diaphoretic, diuretic, mild cathartic, and emetic, as dose increases; also, used in antiseptic and discutient fomentations or gargles. Its effects are attributable to the "coldness of its solution," and to the stimulation produced by the salt. [1,2,15,23,29]

AMMONIAE ACETATAE, AQUA: Ammonium acetate. Aperient, diaphoretic, and febrifuge. [15,23] Also see SPIRITS OF MINDERERUS.

AMMONIAE, AQUA (or SPIRITUS SALIS AMMONIACI): An aqueous solution of SAL AMMONIAC. Tonic, antacid, stomachic, and diaphoretic when given internally;

rubefacient when applied topically. [23] Now defined as 28–29% ammonia in water.

AMMONIAE AROMATICUS, SPIRITUS: "Aromatic spirits of ammonia," made of SPIRITUS AMMONIAE, ROSMARINUS, and oil of LIMON. Now made with ammonium carbonate (see HARTSHORN, def. no. 3), ammonia water, OL LIMONI, OL LAVENDULLA, oil of NUTMEG, alcohol, and water; used as smelling salts.

AMMONIAE COMPOSITUS, SPIRITUS: "Compound spirits of ammonia," same as SPIRITUS AMMONIAE AROMATICUS.

AMMONIAE FOETIDUS, SPIRITUS: "Fetid spirits of ammonia," made of SAL AMMONIAC and ASAFOETIDA in alcohol. Antihysteric. [15]

AMMONIAE FORTIOR, LIQUOR: Strong aqueous solution of ammonia (i.e., ammonium hydroxide) at specific gravity 0.882, introduced by 1836. Used in liniments as a rubefacient, vesicant, and caustic. [29]

AMMONIAE, LINIMENTUM: Ammonia water and OL OLIVA. Used as an antiseptic gargle, a warm tonic, or, when applied externally, as a diaphoretic. [1,15,23]

AMMONIAE, MURIAS: Same as SAL AMMONIAC.

AMMONIAE, SPIRITUS: A mixture of SAL AMMONIAC and LIXIVA that was distilled (producing ammonia and potassium chloride) and added to alcohol. Used as a menstruum, and as a diaphoretic, nerve stimulant, and febrifuge. [2,15]

AMMONIAE SUCCINATUS, SPIRITUS: "Amberized spirits of ammonia." Alcohol extract of ammonia and OL SUCCINUM. Used as smelling salts, and as a snakebite remedy. [15]

AMMONIA PRAEPARATA: Ammonium carbonate (although calcium carbonate was meant in some pharmacopoeias). Tonic, diaphoretic, antispasmodic, antacid, antiseptic, antihysteric, and a remedy for venomous snake bites. [15,23,30] Now the principal ingredient of smelling salts (see AMMONIAE AROMATICUS).

AMMONIARETI CUPRI, PILULE: "Pill of ammoniated copper," made with CUPRUM AMMONIACUM, AMMONIAE PRAEPARATA, and MICA PANIO. Antispasmodic, antiepileptic. [23]

AMMONIATUM, OLEUM: Same as LINIMENTUM AMMONIAE.

AMOMUM GRANUM PARADISI: See GRANA PARADISI.

AMOMUM REPENS: "Freshening shrub," same as CARDAMOMUM MINUS.

AMOMUM ZINGIBER: Same as ZINGIBER.

AMYGDALAE, LAC: "Almond milk," oil from kernels of sweet or Jordan almonds, *Prunus amygdalus dulcis*, added to sugar water. Diluent; also used as an emollient and demulcent laxative, and to counteract CANTHARIS or other irritating medicines. [15,29]

AMYGDALA, OL: Oil of bitter almonds, from *Prunus amygdalus amara* or, sometimes, from sweet almonds, *P. amygdalus dulcis*. Used internally as a sedative, antispasmodic, and expectorant, and externally as an emollient and to relax tense muscles. Said to be poisonous to dogs but not to men. [15,29] Its poisonous principle, hydrocyanic acid, had been identified by Swedish chemist Karl Wilhelm Scheele in 1782, and was isolated from bitter almonds by German chemist Jeremiah Benjamin Richter in 1802.

AMYGDALUS COMMUNIS: Sweet almond; see LAC AMYGDALAE and OL AMYGDALAE.

AMYGDALUS PERSICA: Same as PERSICA.

AMYLUM: 1) Wheat starch; see TRITICUM. Made into a mucilage used in enemas for patients with diarrhea. 2) Occasionally, same as MARANTA ARUNDIACEA.

Anacollemata: Medicines applied to forehead and temples to arrest movement of humors down over the eye.

ANACYCLUS PYRETHRUM: See PYRETHRUM.

ANAGALLIS: Pimpernel, *Anagallis arvensis*. Stomachic, antispasmodic.

Analeptic: A strengthening, restorative medicine.

ANAMIRTA COCCULUS: See COCCULUS.

ANCHUSA: See BUGLOSSUM.

ANDERSON'S [SCOTS] PILLS: First described, as "Grana Angelica" ("Angelic Grains"), by Patrick Anderson in 1635. His daughter sold the formula, which included ALOES, JALAP, GAMBOGE, and ANISUM, to Dr. Thomas Weir of Edinburgh, who patented the cathartic panacea in 1687. Although several competitors sold the same product, they often added RHEI, GUM MASTIC, and various stomachics. By the early 19th century the pills were made with ALOES, JALAP, and OL ANISI. [14]

ANDROMACHE: Same as THERIAC.

ANDROSAEMIFOLIUM: See APOCYNUM ANDROSAEMIFOLIUM.

ANEMONE, MEADOW: See PULSATILLA NIGRICANS.

ANETHUM FOENICULUM: Same as FOENICULUM DULCE.

ANETHUM [GRAVEOLENS]: Seed of dill, *Anethum graveolens*. An aromatic carminative. [15,23,29]

ANGELICA: All parts of *Angelica archangelica* or, in the U.S., *A. sylvestris* or Alexander's angelica, *A. atropurpurea*. Delicate aromatic aperient, tonic, and carminative. [15,29]

ANGELICA, PILULE: "Angelic pill," same as FRANKFURT PILL.

ANGELICA TREE: Same as ARALIA SPINOSA.

ANGUSTURA, CORTEX: Bark of *Cusparia angustura*, introduced from Venezuela to Britain in 1788 or *Galipea officinalis*. Tonic, carminative, digestive, cathartic, and antidiarrheal. [1,2,23,29,30]

Anhaltina: Remedies that ease respiration.

ANIMA HEPATIS: Same as FERRUM VITRIOLATUM.

ANIMAL OIL: A black oil expressed from fresh HARTSHORN (or other horns). Invented in the early 18th century by German physician and alchemist Johann Konrad Dippel. Anodyne, antispasmodic, and diaphoretic. [15]

ANISE: See ANISUM.

ANISI COMPOSITUS, SPIRITUS: "Compound spirits of anise," made of SEMINA ANISUM and ANGELICA seed in alcohol. Antispasmodic for colic. [15]

ANISUM: Seeds, or oil from seeds, of anise, *Pimpinella anisum*. Tonic, pectoral, and carminative; lactagogue. [2,15,23,29] Contains anethole, which stimulates intestinal activity.

Anodyne: An analgesic, usually one made with OPIUM.

ANODYNE BALSAM: Same as LINAMENTUM OPIATUM.

ANODYNE NECKLACE: Its beads were made of PAEONIA wood. Used to cure epilepsy, assuage the pain of cutting teeth, and to protect pregnant women.

Antacid: An alkaline or earthy substance that neutralizes stomach acids. Used for, e.g., dyspepsia and diarrhea. Also see Absorbent.

ANTE CIBUM, PILULE: A stomachic pill made with ALOES, to be taken preprandially.

Anthelminthic: An agent that expels worms from the intestinal canal, because of the roughness of the drug particles, its cathartic action, or, in a few cases, because of a specific toxic effect on the worms themselves.

ANTHEMIS COTULA: See COTULA FOETIDA.

ANTHEMIS [NOBILIS]: Same as CHAMAEMELUM.

ANTHRISCUS: See CEREFOLIUM.

Antianginal: A remedy for painful spasmodic suffocation, as in, e.g., croup or asthma; not a remedy for angina pectoris.

Anticephalic: A head ache remedy.

Antiepileptic: A medicine used in treating epilepsy (however, most convulsions were not caused by what would be diagnosed as epilepsy today, but by high fevers).

Antihectic: A medicine used to treat hectic fevers, which increase in the evening and after eating, and are typically associated with flushed cheeks, especially in consumption.

ANTIHECTICUM POTERII: "Antihectic of Poterius." Same as DIAPHORETICUM JOVIALE. Named for 16th–century French Paracelsian physician Pierre de la Poterie.

Antihypochondriaca: Remedies for hypochondriacal (i.e., with manifestations in the abdomen) melancholy.

Antihysteric: A drug used to treat "hypochondriasis," also called "the spleen," "vapours," "melancholy," and, in women, "the hysteric disease." Whatever its cause, by the late 18th century hysteria was thought to result from "a laxity of the fibres, or flatulence, exciting spasms in various parts of the body, and a variety of other symptoms." [11] Antihysteric was often used as a synonym for Emmenagogue. Also see PESSARIES.

ANTIHYSTERIC PLASTER: Made of LITHARGE, ASAFOETIDA, GALBANUM, and CERA FLAVA, applied to the umbilical region. Antispasmodic, expectorant, emmenagogue, and anthelminthic. [2,15]

Anti-icteric: A medicine used in the treatment of jaundice (icterus).

Antilienteric: An antidiarrheal drug.

Antilithic: A drug that prevents or destroys kidney or bladder stones. Also see Lithontriptic.

Antilyssus, Pulvis: A remedy for rabies.

ANTIMONIAL AETHIOPS: A diaphoretic made with AETHIOPS MINERALIS, HYDRARGYRUS, and ANTIMONIUM CRUDUM. [12]

ANTIMONIALIS, PULVIS: ANTIMONIUM CRUDUM (57 parts) burned with HARTSHORN (43 parts); commonly called JAMES'S POWDER, although its formula is also commonly given as one part of antimony trioxide (Sb_2O_3) and two parts of calcium dibasic phosphate ($CaHPO_4 \cdot 2H_2O$). Diaphoretic febrifuge; vomiting and catharsis follow high doses. [15,23,30]

ANTIMONII, BUTYRUM: "Butter of antimony;" antimony trichloride but thought to be same as ANTIMONIUM MURIATUM.

ANTIMONII, CROCUS: Antimony oxide; used for preparing other antimony salts. [2,15] Actually a mixture of antimony oxide (Sb_2O_5) and antimony oxysulfite.

ANTIMONII, ESSENTIA: Same as ANTIMONIUM VITRIFICATUM.

ANTIMONII ET POTASSAE TARTRAS: Same as ANTIMONIUM TARTARISATUM.

ANTIMONII, VINUM: ANTIMONY in Spanish white wine. Alterative and diaphoretic in low doses; diuretic and cathartic at higher doses; violently emetic at even larger doses that are suitable for "some maniacal and apoplectic cases." [15]

ANTIMONII VITRUM CERATUM: "Cerated glass of antimony," a powder made by mixing ANTIMONIUM VITRIFICATUM with CERA FLAVA. Cathartic, emetic, and sometimes diaphoretic. [15,23] Also see CHYLISTA.

ANTIMONIUM [CRUDUM]: Native ore of antimony, consisting chiefly of the trisulfide. According to medical mythology, antimony was discovered by Basil Valentine, a 15th-century monk at Erfurt, but it was probably discovered by Johann Tholde in 1604. Emetic, cathartic, tonic, diaphoretic, and febrifuge, but usually prescribed in this form only for skin eruptions. [1,2,23]

ANTIMONIUM CALCAREO PHOSPHORATUM: Same as PULVIS ANTIMONIALIS.

ANTIMONIUM CALCINATUM: Antimony nitrate. Weakly diaphoretic and emetic. [15]

ANTIMONIUM DIAGREDIATUM: A mixture of ANTIMONIUM and SCAMMONIUM.

ANTIMONIUM DIAPHORETICUM LOTUM or NITRATUM: Same as ANTIMONIUM CALCINATUM.

ANTIMONIUM MURIATUM: Thought to be antimony

chloride, but actually the oxychloride. Caustic, but used chiefly only in manufacturing ANTIMONIUM TARTARISATUM.

ANTIMONIUM TARTARISATUM: Tartar emetic, or antimony potassium tartrate, the most frequently prescribed of all antimony compounds. Introduced by Adrian Mynsicht of Mecklenberg by 1631 (although Paracelsus had prepared and prescribed it a century earlier). Sedates the circulation, while it excites the secretions. Diaphoretic, cathartic, and expectorant at low doses, and emetic at high doses. Sometimes applied topically because it has a counterirritant effect like that of CANTHARIS. [1,2,15,23,29,30]

ANTIMONIUM USTUM CUM NITRO: Same as ANTIMONIUM CALCINATUM.

ANTIMONIUM VITRIFICATUM: "Glass of antimony," prepared by melting antimony ore until no more sulfur escapes. Emetic, but too potent for routine internal administration; used chiefly in preparing other antimonials, especially ANTIMONII VITRUM CERATUM. [15,23]

ANTIMONY: See ANTIMONIUM.

ANTIMONY SULPHATE: Same as VITRIOL ANTIMONIUM.

Antiphlogistic: A medicine used to neutralize fevers. The Greek word *phlogiston*, which referred to fire or "a flame principle," represented a material component of all combustible substances. In 1669, Robert Boyle (1627-1691) had showed that air is necessary for the maintenance of both animal life and combustion. Nevertheless, at about the same time, two German physicians and chemists, Johann Joachim Becher (1635-82) and Georg Ernst Stahl (1660-1734), hypothesized that when a candle burns within a closed space, it gives off phlogiston, so that the air around it becomes "phlogisticated" and can no longer support combustion. In 1771-1774, English clergyman and chemist Joseph Priestley (1733-1804) showed that "phlogisticated air" can be restored, or "dephlogisticated," by green plants, and that "dephlogisticated air" is about one-fifth of atmospheric air. Thus, the phlogiston theory held that substances burn as phlogiston escapes from them. Because clinically apparent inflammations were warm to the touch, and often made the patient feel warm, such illnesses—fevers—were interpreted in terms of phlogiston, and were treated with drugs thought to counteract the calorigenic effect associated with it.

Much earlier, Flemish physician and chemist Jan Baptista van Helmont (1577-1644) had discovered how to produce "gas carbonum" (carbon dioxide) by burning charcoal. In 1754, Dr. Joseph Black (1728-1799) of Edinburgh found that slaked lime (calcium hydroxide, $Ca(OH)_2$), loses weight when it is burned to quicklime (calcium oxide, CaO). This contradicted Stahl's phlogiston theory, which dictated that lime should increase in weight when it is converted to quicklime. Then in 1757 Black also found that the loss of weight is attributable to the loss of a specific gas that he identified as van Helmont's "gas carbonum," and he renamed it "fixed air."

In 1774, French chemist Antoine-Laurent Lavoisier (1743-94) found that oxygen was absorbed by metals when they formed "calces" (i.e., oxides). Although Priestley had shown, in 1772, that animals remove some vital substance from the air when they breathe, he continued to accept the existence of phlogiston. In 1780, Lavoisier went on to demonstrate the role of Priestley's "vital air"—oxygen—in both respiration and combustion. That is, he found that the production of animal heat was analogous to slow combustion, and that inspired air is converted, within the body, to "fixed air."

Still, despite the accumulating evidence that phlogiston did not exist, remedies used in the treatment of inflammations and fevers continued to be described as "antiphlogistic" into the 19th century. Dr. William Cullen of Edinburgh summarized this typical first line of defense against fevers as the purposeful avoidance or moderation of the usual irritations that may affect the body. He said that an effective "antiphlogistic regimen" should include avoidance of: 1) external heat, exercise, thirst, and excessive food and mental activity, through rest and with a "low" DIET; 2) corruption of humors in the stomach, by administering emetics, acids, or diluents; 3) fecal retention, by administering cathartics and enemas; and 4) acrimony of body fluids, by administering diaphoretics and antiseptics. The use of other drugs, or techniques such as BLEEDING and BLISTERS, was dictated by the particular species of fever involved, as well as by its severity; such therapies were supplementary components of the antiphlogistic regimen, and depended on the physician's assessment of each patient's special needs. [See Cullen's *First Lines of the Practice of Physic*, new ed., 4 vols. (Edinburgh and London, 1789), I, 255-258; also see ref. 1, pp. 177-225, and 46.]

Antiphthisica: Remedies for phthisis, i.e., consumption (now recognized as tuberculosis in most—but not all—cases).

ANTIPHTHISICA, TINCTURA: Tincture of CERUSSA ACETATA, used in consumption to inhibit sweating.

ANTIPHTHISICUS HALY, PULVIS: See HALY, POWDER OF.

Antipodagrica: Remedies for gout.

ANTIPSORICUM, UNGUENTUM: Ointment made with SULPHUR, AXUNGUENTUM PORCINUM, and oil of LIMON or oil of LAVENDULA. A remedy for itch. [15]

Antipyretic: A fever remedy.

Antirheumatic: A drug that dissolves rheum (i.e., blockage of the nostrils associated with coughing and sneezing); often also applied to Diaphoretics.

Antiscorbutic: A medicine used in the treatment of scurvy ("scorbutus"). Also see LIMON.

Antiseptic: A drug that prevents putrefaction ("sepsis").

Antispasmodic: A drug that reduces spasms, including those of the cardiovascular system (as manifested by a rapid pulse), but without causing insensibility or otherwise affecting the brain (as narcotics do).

Antitussive: A cough remedy.

Aperient: A weak cathartic.

APIUM: Smallage, or wild celery, *Apium graveolens*. Aromatic, aperient, and carminative. [15]

Apocrustica: Astringent remedies.

APOCYNUM [ANDROSAEMIFOLIUM]: Root of spreading dogbane, *Apocynum androsaemifolium*. Tonic and stomachic at low doses, emetic at high doses. [29,30]

APOCYNUM CANNABINUM: Root of dog's bane, or Indian hemp, *Apocynum cannabinum*. Strong emetic and cathartic; also, diuretic, diaphoretic, and expectorant. [29]

Apodagritica: Remedies that stop the involuntary flow of tears from the eyes.

Apophlegmatismus: A remedy that, when chewed, stimulates salivation.

APOSTOLORUM, UNGUENTUM: "Ointment of the Apostles," made of TEREBINTHA, CERA ALBA, WHITE LEAD, MYRHHA, OPOPANAX, and seven other ingredients, hence the drug's name (in which the word Apostles stands for the number 12).

Apothecary Weights: See Measurement.

Apothems: Same as Apozema.

Apozema (or Apozemata): Strong infusions or decoctions of vegetable drugs. [2]

APPLE OF PERU: Same as STRAMONIUM.

Aquae [Distillatae or Stillatitiae]: Distilled aqueous extracts of plant materials, or simple solutions of inorganic compounds. Some were simply decanted from infusions, and no heat at all was applied to others.

AQUILA ALBA: "White eagle," same as CALOMEL.

ARABICA, EMULSIO: Same as LAC AMYGDALAE.

ARABICAE, PILULE: Pill made of ALOES, BRYONIA, MYROBALANI, CITRUS, and 11 other ingredients.

ARABIC, GUM: Extract of *Acacia senegal* (or *A. verek*). Demulcent and sedative. [1,2,15,23,29] Also used as a cheap substitute for ACACIA VERA. Still used as a menstruum and demulcent.

Araeotica: Remedies that rarefy and thin the humors and open the pores of the body, e.g., Diaphoretics.

ARALIA [NUDICAULIS]: Wild or false sarsaparilla, *Aralia nudicaulis*. Mild diaphoretic. Also see SARSAPARILLA.

ARALIA SPINOSA: Twigs from toothache tree, *Zanthoxylum americanum* (in southern U.S., *Z. clava-Hercules*; see XANTHOXYLUM CLAVUS HERCULES). Diaphoretic; toothache remedy; and, antispasmodic for colic. [2,23,29] Emetic and cathartic. [30] Contains the alkaloid berberine; see BERBERIS.

ARBUTUS UVA URSI: See UVA URSI.

ARCAEI, LINIMENTUM: "Astringent liniment," made with ELEMI, OL TEREBINTHA, OL OLIVA, and OVIS. For cleaning and "digesting" wounds. [15]

Arcanum: Paracelsian term for a compound remedy.

ARCANUM CORALLINUM: "Coral secret." See CORALLIUM RUBRUM, def. no. 2.

ARCANUM DUPLICATUM: "Double secret," same as KALI SULPHURATUM.

ARCTIUM LAPPA: Same as BARDANA.

ARCTOSTAPHYLUS UVA-URSI: See UVA URSI.

ARECA: Same as CATECHU.

ARGEMONE MEXICANA: Yellow juice of prickly poppy, or yellow thistle, *Argemone* spp. Detersive, resolvent, narcotic, diaphoretic, and antidiarrheal. [23]

ARGENTUM: Silver.

ARGENTUM NITRATUM: Silver nitrate. Used chiefly as a caustic for warts, fungating wounds, etc., but sometimes as a gentle cathartic, tonic, astringent, antihelminthic, and antianginal. [15,23,30] Still placed in the eyes of newborns to prevent gonococcal ophthalmia.

ARGENTUM VIVUM: Elemental mercury ("quicksilver").

ARGIL: Same as ALUM.

ARISTOLOCHIA [LONGA]: Birthwort, any of several vines of the genus *Aristolochia*. Heating, tonic, diuretic, diaphoretic, and to suppress menses; applied externally as a styptic. [15] Also see SERPENTARIA.

ARMARIUM, UNGUENTUM: "Weapon ointment," same as SYMPATHETIC OINTMENT.

ARMENIAN BOLE (also, BOLUS ARMENUS, BOLE ARMENIC, BOLE ARMENIAK, etc.): A bright red BOLUS that effervesces with acids; contains aluminum silicate and FERRI RUBIGO. Astringent, hemostatic, absorbent.

ARMORACIA: Same as RAPHANUS RUSTICANUS.

ARNICA MONTANA: Leaves of leopard's bane, *Arnica montana*. Introduced to medical practice in Germany in 1712, and popularized as a substitute for CINCHONA by Dr. Henry Joseph Collin of Vienna in 1773. Once used to inhibit accumulations of edema fluid, it was later promoted as a tonic for paralysis, and as an antispasmodic febrifuge; also, narcotic, diuretic, diaphoretic, and emmenagogue, and, in high doses, cathartic and emetic. [1,15,29]

Aromatic: A spicy drug.

AROMATICA, CONFECTIO: Same as formula no. 2 for AROMATIC ELECTUARY.

AROMATICA, PILULE: Nearly the same as PILULE ALOES CUM GUAIACUM.

AROMATICA, TINCTURA: Alcohol extract of CINNAMOMUM, CARDAMOMUM MINUS, PIPER LONGUM, and ANGELICA. A mild tonic. [1]

AROMATIC ELECTUARY: Several formulations, including: 1) CINNAMOMUM, CARDAMOMUM MINUS, ZINGIBER, and syrup of CORTEX AURANTIUM; the same ingredients were used in AQUA CARDIACA [1,2]; 2) ZEDOARIA, CROCUS, CANCER LAPILLI, CINNAMOMUM, NUTMEG, CARYOPHYLLUS, and CARDAMOMUM MINUS [15]; 3) PULVIS AROMA-

TICA and syrup of CORTEX AURANTIUM [15]. A warm cordial and cardiac drug.

AROMATIC PILL: Same as AROMATIC ELECTUARY, def. no. 1.

AROMATIC SPECIES: Same as PULVIS AROMATICUS.

AROMATICUS ACETATUS, SPIRITUS: Same as SPIRITUS AROMATICUS but with vinegar (ACETUM) added.

AROMATICUS, PULVIS: Aromatic powder made of CINNAMOMUM, CARDAMOMUM MINUS, ZINGIBER, and PIPER LONGUM. Stomachic; visceral tonic. [15]

AROMATICUS, SPIRITUS: Made with ROSMARINUS, MILLEFOLIUM, THYMUS, and PROOF SPIRIT. Properties like those of HUNGARY WATER, but used chiefly as a prophylactic fumigant, "to destroy the influence of febrile contagions." [15]

ARQUEBUSADE WATER: A weak distillate of as many as 24 antiseptic and aromatic plants designed to treat wounds made by the arquebus, a 16th-century gun.

ARROWROOT: See MARANTA ARUDINACEA.

ARSENICALIS, LIQUOR: Same as SOLUTIO MINERALIS ARSENICI.

ARSENICI, SOLUTIO MINERALIS: Water solution of WHITE ARSENIC and LIXIVA, best known as FOWLER'S SOLUTION; spirit of LAVENDULA was sometimes added. Used chiefly as a tonic diaphoretic and alterative, especially for intermittent fevers. [1,15,23] The modern formula includes the same ingredients (as arsenic trioxide, potassium bicarbonate, alcohol, and tincture of lavender).

ARSENICUM: Arsenic; most widely used as SOLUTIO MINERALIS ARSENICI. Usually a violent, and highly inflammatory, poison; small doses produce tremors and fluctuating fever. Also used as a topical corrosive for cancer in a secret remedy prepared by the Plunkett family in Ireland, and as an internal remedy for cancer and intermittent fevers. Antidotes include milk, oily liquors, acids (e.g., ACETUM), and KALI SULPHURATUM. [15]

ARSENIC, WHITE: Arsenic trioxide. A violent corrosive poison, but used medically in SOLUTIO MINERALIS ARSENICI. [29]

ARSENIOSUM, ACIDUM: Same as WHITE ARSENIC.

ARTEMISIA: Usually, leaves of mugwort, *Artemisia vulgaris.*

Emmenagogue and antihysteric. [15] However, also see ABROTANUM, ABSINTHUM entries, and SANTONICUM.

ARTHANITA: Root of sowbread, *Cyclamen europaeum*. Errhine, but sometimes taken internally as a cathartic, detergent, and aperient, or used in cataplasms. [15]

Arthritica: Remedies for joint pains.

ARTICHOKE: See CINARA.

ARUM AMERICANUM: Root and seeds of skunk cabbage, *Symplocarpus foetidus*. Antispasmodic and narcotic, especially in asthma, labor, and rheumatism. [23,29,30]

ARUM [MACULATUM]: Root of cuckoopint, dragon root, or wake robin, *Arum maculatum*. Tonic, expectorant, and diaphoretic. [15,23,29]

ARUM TRIPHYLLUM: Root of Indian turnip, or small jack-in-the-pulpit, *Arum triphyllum*. Antispasmodic, for asthma and violent coughing. [23]

ASA DULCIS: Same as BENZOIN.

AS[S]AFOETIDA (or ASSA F[O]ETIDA): Gum-resin of root of *Ferula assafoetida*. Antispasmodic, antihysteric, expectorant, emmenagogue, diuretic, diaphoretic, weak laxative, and anthelminthic. [1,2,15,23,29,30]

ASAFOETIDAE COMPOSITAE, PILULE: "Compound pills of ASAFOETIDA," mixed with GALBANUM, MYRRH, and OL SUCCINI. Antihysteric and emmenagogue. [23]

ASAFOETIDAE, LAC: "Milk of asafoetida," an emulsion of ASAFOETIDA in water. Antihysteric; given by mouth or rectum. [15]

ASARABACCA: See ASARUM.

ASARI COMPOSITUS, PULVIS: "Compound powder of asarabacca," made with ASARUM (def. no. 1), MAJORANA, MARUM SYRIACUM, and LAVENDULA. Powerful errhine, for headache and ophthalmia. [15]

ASARUM: 1) In Europe, leaves of asarabacca, or hazelwort, *Asarum europaeum*. Used chiefly as an errhine, but also for its emetic, cathartic, diuretic, diaphoretic, and emmenagogue properties. [15,29] 2) In U.S., root of wild ginger, or Canada snakeroot, *Asarum canadense*. Tonic and diaphoretic. [29,30]

ASCLEPIAS DECUMBENS: Root of butterfly weed or pleurisy root, *Asclepias tuberosa*. Diaphoretic, expectorant, and febrifuge; mild cathartic and carminative. [23,30]

ASCLEPIAS INCARNATA: Root of swamp, or flesh-colored, milkweed, *Asclepias incarnata.* Expectorant, diaphoretic, and diuretic; in large doses, cathartic. [29,30]

ASCLEPIAS SYRIACA: Root of common milkweed, *Asclepias syriaca.* Anodyne, expectorant, antispasmodic, and antitussive. [29,30]

ASCLEPIAS TUBEROSA: Same as ASCLEPIAS DECUMBENS.

ASH: See FRAXINUS.

ASPARAGUS: Roots and shoots of *Asparagus officinalis.* Diuretic, aperient, and deobstruent, but not dependable. [15]

ASSAIERET, PILULE: "Cleansing pill," a cathartic and stomachic preparation made with HIERA PICRA, MASTICHE, CITRUS, MYROBALANS, ALOES, and STECHAS.

ASTACUS: See CANCRORUM LAPILLI.

ASTHMATICUS, ELIXIR: Usually, same as TINCTURA OPII CAMPHORATA, but sometimes means LAUDANUM. [1,2,15]

ASTRAGALUS TRAGACANTHA (or CRETICUS): See GUM TRAGACANTH.

Astringent: A drug that strengthens the body when it is relaxed, or that diminishes the excessive evacuations (e.g., hemorrhage, menorrhagia, hemoptysis, diarrhea, excessive sweating, and the polyuria of diabetes mellitus) that may accompany debilities and fevers, by condensing or contracting the tissues of which the vessels are formed. External astringents, or styptics, contract broken or ulcerated skin.

Asyncriticum, Medicamentum: "An unparalleled remedy."

ATHANATIA MAGNA: Literally, "great antidote to death." A strong preparation of OPIUM prescribed as an antihysteric and to induce sleep.

ATRIPLEX FOETIDA: Leaves of stinking orach, *Chenopodium vulvaria.* Antihysteric. [15]

ATROPA BELLADONNA: See BELLADONNA.

ATROPA MANDRAGORA: See MANDRAGORA, def. no. 1.

Attenuantia: Remedies that penetrate, rarefy, and divide the humors into smaller parts.

ATTRAHENS, EMPLASTRUM: "Attracting plaster," same as EMPLASTRUM CERAE COMPOSITUM.

AURANTIUM [HISPALENSE] CORTEX: Rind of Spanish, or Seville, orange, *Citrus aurantium*. Tonic, refrigerant, antispasmodic, stomachic, carminative, antiseptic, and antiscorbutic; but used chiefly for flavoring. [2,15,23,29]

AUREA ALEXANDRINA: A complex drug made with AURUM and OPIUM attributed to a Dr. Alexander.

AUREUM UNGUENTUM: A gold-colored ointment.

AURUM: Gold. Rarely used in medicines, chiefly as an antispasmodic; sometimes recommended as an antivenereal. [15,23,30] Occasionally used today in treatment of severe rheumatoid arthritis.

AURUM POTABILE: "Potable gold," a solution of gold in wine vinegar, was originally a concept of the 16th–century Paracelsian physician Francis Anthony of London, but by the late 18th century it had become decoction of LENTISCUS.

AVENA [SATIVA]: Oats, *Avena sativa*. Used chiefly for their nutritive value, although oatmeal's mucilaginous property was also used for respiratory tract inflammations and for producing a gentle catharsis. [15]

AVENA FARINA: Oatmeal.

AVENS: See CARYOPHYLLATA and GEUM RIVALE.

Avoirdupois Weights: See Measurement.

AXUNGUENTUM PORCINUM: "Pork grease." Lard (hog fat), used chiefly as an emollient in ointments. [1]

AZEDARACH: Same as MELIA AZEDARACH.

AZYMUS, PANIS: "Unleavened bread," used to coat certain pills and boluses.

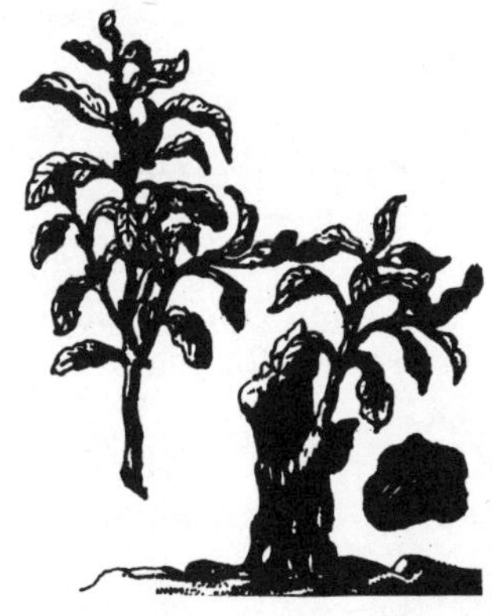

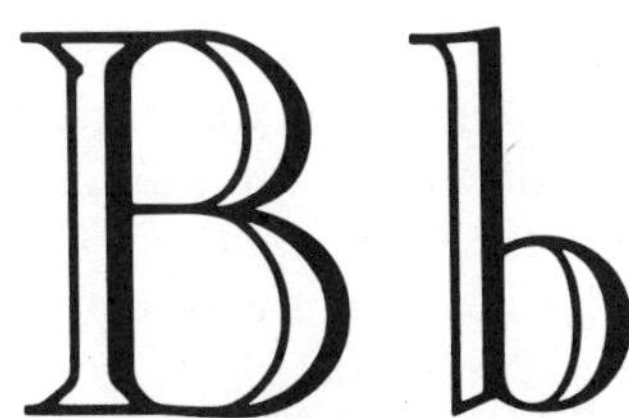

Benjamin tree

BACHE'S (or BACHER'S) PILL: Same as BECHER'S TONIC PILL.

BALDMONEY: See MEUM.

BALLSTON MINERAL WATER: A leading American mineral water from New York state in the early 19th century, it was being manufactured by 1809. One analysis showed that it contained FIXED AIR (in a ratio of 3:1 to the volume of water), SAL MURIATICUS, CRETA, MURIATIS CALCIS, magnesium chloride, and, as its most important ingredient, FERRI RUBIGO. Prescribed as a gentle cathartic, diuretic, and general tonic. [ref. 23, pp. 568-572]

BALM GENTLE (or BALM MINT): See MELISSA.

BALM-WATER, COMPOUND: Same as AQUA CARMELITANA.

Balnea: Medicated baths.

BALSAM DROPS: Probably usually same as BALSAMUM CANADENSE.

Balsamic: A softening, restoring, healing, and cleansing medicine.

BALSAMITA: Leaves of costumary, *Chrysanthemum* (or *Tan-*

acetum) balsamita. Ineffectual antihysteric, and an antidote to OPIUM. [15]

BANEBERRY, RED: See ACTEA SPICATA.

BAPTISIA TINCTORIA: See SOPHORA TINCTORIA.

BARBERRY: See BERBERIS.

BARDANA: Root or seeds of burdock, *Arctium lappa.* Aperient, diuretic, diaphoretic, and blood purifier; seeds are diuretic. [15,23,29]

BARICIS: Barium sulfate. Tonic, diaphoretic, diuretic, and escharotic. [2]

BARILLA: Natron, a naturally–occurring mixture of sodium carbonate and sodium bicarbonate, with sodium chloride and sodium sulfate as impurities. After a process for manufacturing the carbonate was discovered in 1784, the word barilla was sometimes used to mean CARBONAS SODAE. Native barilla was used chiefly for preparing other compounds.

BARK: When used alone, same as CINCHONA.

BARK, PERUVIAN: Same as CINCHONA.

BARK VAN SWIETEN: Same as CINCHONA.

BARLEY: See HORDEUM.

BAROSMA: See BUCHU.

BARYTA (or BARYTES): Heavy earth, principally barium sulfate. Used by miners as a rat poison, and by physicians to stimulate all excretions, but chiefly to prepare MURIAS BARYTAE.

BARYTES, MURIATE OF: Same as MURIAS BARYTAE.

BASILICON OINTMENT: "Sovereign ointment." One recipe included ABIES, AXUNGUENTUM PORCINUM, CERA FLAVA, and sometimes OL OLIVA. Emollient. [2,15] Also see YELLOW BASILICON.

BASTARD SAFFRON THISTLE: See CARTHAMUS.

BATEANA, AQUA ALUMINOSA: "Bate's aluminated water," devised by Dr. William Bate of London in mid–17th century. Same as AQUA ALUMINIS COMPOSITA.

BATEMAN'S PECTORAL DROPS: A proprietary remedy sold as early as 1721, and patented by businessman Benjamin Okell in 1723, as a diaphoretic, diuretic, lithontriptic, and antihysteric. Later formulations, by various manufacturers, contained 0.1 to 7.0% OPIUM, although other ingredients (e.g., RHEI, CAMPHOR, CATECHU, ANISUM, COCHINEAL, and ALCOHOL) were included at various times. [13,14]

BATE'S HYSTERIC JULEP: See HYSTERIC JULEP WITH MUSK. Introduced in the mid-17th century by Dr. William Bate of London.

BATE'S PACIFICK PILL: see PACIFICK PILL.

BAYBERRY: See LAURUS.

BDELLIUM: Gum from a *Balsamodendron* species. Used in plasters, and as a diaphoretic, diuretic, and emmenagogue. [15]

BEARBERRY: See UVA URSI.

BEAR'S FOOT: See HELLEBORASTER.

BECCABUNGA: Brooklime, or speedwell, *Veronica becabunga*. Bitter aromatic, mild stimulant, detergent, and antiscorbutic. [15]

BECHER'S TONIC PILL: Made of HELLEBORUS NIGER, MYRRH, and CARDUUS BENEDICTUS. Cathartic, diuretic, and tonic remedy devised by German physician Johann Joachim Becher of London; promoted in late 18th-century for dropsy. [15,29]

BECHICI TROCHISCI: Literally, "TUSSILAGO troches," which were prescribed for respiratory ailments. However, TUSSILAGO had disappeared from their formulas by the late 18th century: e.g., Troschici bechici albi ("White Pectoral Troches," made with GUM ARABIC), Troschici bechici nigri ("Black Pectoral Troches," made with GLYCERRHIZA and GUM ARABIC), and Trochisci bechici cum opio ("Pectoral Troches with Opium," made with GLYCERRHIZA and OPIUM).

BELLADONNA: Leaves of deadly nightshade, *Atropa belladonna*. Long known as a poison, belladonna was probably introduced to medical practice about 1150, but certainly by 1526, in the Parisian *Grand Herbier* of Pierre Sergent. Administered internally as a strong narcotic, diuretic, diaphoretic, and sialagogue; its side effects include dry mouth, dysphagia, "anxiety" in the chest, delirium, flushing, mydriasis, severe abdominal pain, convulsions, and coma. Applied externally as a sedative, as an anodyne, to promote suppuration, and as a discutient in cancer. Also used to dilate the pupil in preparation for cataract extraction. [1,15,23,29,30] Now known to contain the antimuscarinic alkaloid atropine, isolated from the leaves in 1833 by Philipp Lorenz Geiger and Germain Henri Hess of Heidelberg. The leaves contain 0.44 to 0.48% atropine, as well as hyoscyamine.

BENEDICTA LAXATIVA: "Blessed laxative," a strong cathartic, antihysteric, and carminative electuary, made with SENNA, TAMARINDUS, CASSIA, PRUNUS GALLICA, CORIANDRUM, GLYCERRHIZA, and sugar.

BENEDICTUM, VINUM: "Blessed wine," a solution of ANTIMONIUM VITRIFICATUM in wine. Prescribed as an attenuant, deobstruent, alterative, diaphoretic, diuretic, and, in large doses, as an emetic. [20]

BENJAMIN TREE: See BENZOIN.

BENNE: See SESAMUM ORIENTALE.

BENZOIN [FLOWERS OF]: Benzoic acid (identified by 1617), extracted from the benjamin tree, *Styrax benzoin*. Sometimes called Sal Benzoes, depending on method of preparation. Diaphoretic and expectorant. [2,15,23]

BENZOINI TINCTURA COMPOSITA: Alcohol extract of BENZOIN, BALSAM OF PERU, and hepatic ALOES, sometimes with STYRAX CALAMITA. An external liniment for skin sores and joint pains; taken internally as an intestinal tonic. [15] Also see TURLINGTON'S BALSAM OF LIFE.

BERBERIS: Bark, and berry juice, of barberry, *Berberis vulgaris*. Bark used in jaundice, because it is yellow, and as a cathartic; berries used as a tonic and antiseptic antidiarrheal. [15] An alkaloid, berberine, which has antimicrobial and local anesthetic properties, was isolated from the stems in 1843.

BERKELEY'S TAR WATER: A panacea devised by George Berkeley, Bishop of Cloyne, in 1739-40; 1 qt. tar from PIX LIQUIDA is mixed in 1 gal. water and the supernatant recovered after 3 days. Raises the pulse, and produces diaphoresis, diuresis, and, sometimes, catharsis or emesis. [13,15; also see any edition of Oliver Wendell Holmes' essay on "Homeopathy and its Kindred Delusions"]

BESTUCHEFF'S TINCTURE: Same as GOLDEN DROPS OF GENERAL LA MOTHE.

BETONICA: Leaves and flowers of betony, *Stachys officinalis*. A mild tonic and errhine. The roots are too strongly cathartic and emetic for routine clinical use. [15]

BETTON'S BRITISH OIL: See BRITISH OIL.

BETULA: Juice of birch tree, *Betula alba*. Diuretic in scurvy. [15]

BEYER'S PILL: Same as FRANKFURT PILL.

BEZOAR: 1) Concretion found in the stomach of goats and

related species. A very weak absorbent. [15] 2) In the 17th century, the dried and powdered liver and heart of a snake.

BEZOARTICUM MINERALE: "Mineral bezoar," made of ANTIMONIUM MURIATUM heated with SPIRIT OF NITRE and then reduced to powder and added to SPIRITUS VINOSUS.

BICHLORIDE OF MERCURY: Same as HYDRARGYRUS MURIATUS CORROSIVUS.

BIRCH: See BETULA.

BIRD PEPPER: Same as PIPER INDICUM.

BIRTHWORT: See ARISTOLOCHIA.

BISMUTHUM: Bismuth, especially its oxide. Introduced to the materia medica by Dr. Louis Odier about 1803, as an antispasmodic for abdominal pain. [23,29] Some of its salts are antidiarrheal.

BISTORTA: Root of bistort, or snakeweed, *Polygonum bistorta*. Internal and external astringent. [15,23,29]

Bitter: Usually any bitter-tasting tonic drug that stimulates the appetite (i.e., an appetizer) by virtue of its local irritant action in the stomach.

BITTER APPLE: Same as COLOCYNTHIS.

BITTER INFUSION: Same as INFUSUM AMARUM.

BITTER [PURGING] SALTS [MOULT'S]: Same as MAGNESIA VITRIOLATA.

BITTERSWEET, EUROPEAN: See DULCAMARA.

BITTER WOOD OF SURINAM: Same as QUASSIA.

BITUMEN PETROLEUM: Same as PETROLEUM BARBADENSE.

BLACKBERRY: See RUBUS NIGER.

BLACK COHOSH: See CIMIFUGA.

BLACK DRAUGHT: The original, a strong cathartic preparation introduced in Italy about 1600, was made of SENNA, RIBES, CORIANDRUM, and CREAM OF TARTAR. Over the years its composition was modified until by the late 19th century it was made of MAGNESIA VITRIOLATA or SENNA, sometimes with added MANNA or AMMONIA, but by 1900 it was synonomous with the BLUE PILL. [13]

BLACK DROP: A proprietary remedy introduced about 1700 that contained more OPIUM than most varieties of LAUDANUM; became ACETUM OPII.

BLACK HELLEBORE: See HELLEBORUS NIGER.

BLACK POPLAR: See POPULUS.

BLACK SNAKEROOT: See CIMIFUGA.

BLACKTHORN: See PRUNUS SYLVESTRIS.

BLAUD'S PILLS: Described by Dr. J. Blaud in 1831 as a mixture of FERRUM VITRIOLATUM, GUM ARABIC, and LIXIVA coated with silver [13]; later became "Blaud's mass," which was 36–41% ferrous carbonate (i.e., CARBONAS FERRI) in honey and sugar. Tonic.

BLEEDING: Accomplished by the free flow of blood from a lanced vein; by scarification (12 to 20 small cuts made in the dermis by a set of spring-loaded blades over an area of about 1.5 to 2 square inches); by wet cupping, "cucurbita cum ferro" (in which a glass or other cup from which the air had been evacuated by heat was placed over the scarified area); or, for especially weak patients or for a maximum local effect only, with one or more leeches applied to the affected part of the body (usually the temple, breast, or lateral thorax, but also inside the "mouth, nostrils, or other cavities"), and left on the patient overnight or until they fell off. [1; also see Stephen L. Adams, "The Medicinal Leech: a Page from the Annelids of Internal Medicine," *Annals of Internal Medicine 109* (1988): 399-405]. Although the most common site of venesection was the antecubital vein in the bend of the elbow, it was sometimes accomplished by lancing dorsal foot veins or, in children, by cutting vessels under the tongue.

Dr. William Cullen of Edinburgh noted that "bloodletting is one of the most powerful means of diminishing the activity of the whole body, especially of the sanguiferous system; and it must therefore be the most effectual means of moderating the violence of reaction in fevers," which were often accompanied by a fast pulse. That is, bleeding has a depleting effect which calms the entire body when it is overstimulated. Cullen went on to note that the decision to bleed is made after considering: the nature of the prevailing epidemic; the nature of the remote cause of the patient's disease; the season and climate; the severity of the phlogistic (inflammatory) diathesis present in the patient; his age, vigor, plethoric state, former diseases, and former responses to bleeding; and the appearance of his blood after it has been withdrawn from the body. Finally, Cullen recommended that blood be removed when the body was maximally relaxed, but that bleeding was contraindicated either just before or during the periods of debility that commonly follow the initial inflammatory stages of fevers;

therefore, it was an appropriate early antiphlogistic treatment. [See: William Cullen, *First Lines of the Practice of Physic*, new ed., 4 vols (Edinburgh and London, 1798), I, 194-198.]

"Topical" bleeding techniques (i.e., leeching and cupping) were employed to relieve pain and other symptoms of localized inflammations. That is, the beneficial effects of such techniques were not attributed to any loss of blood mass, as in the case of venesection, but to an effect mediated via the nerve supply to the affected part of the body. Similar reasoning justified the use of CANTHARIS as another method for producing "counter-irritation."

For detailed descriptions of bleeding techniques, and a wealth of illustrations of the tools and techniques employed, see: Audrey Davis and Toby Appel, *Bloodletting Instruments in the National Museum of History and Technology, Smithsonian Studies in History and Technology* No. 41 (Washington, D.C.: Smithsonian Institution Press, 1979).

BLESSED THISTLE: See CARDUUS BENEDICTUS.

BLISTER: see CANTHARIS.

BLOIS, BOLE OF (or, BOLUS BLESENSIS): A pale yellow BOLUS that effervesces strongly with acids.

BLOODROOT: See SANGUINARIA CANADENSIS.

BLUE FLAG: See IRIS PSEUDACORUS.

BLUE OINTMENT: Same as UNGUENTUM HYDRARGYRI.

BLUE PILL: Same as HYDRARGYRUS MURIATUS CORROSIVUS.

BLUE PLASTER: Same as EMPLASTRUM HYDRARGYRI.

BLUE VITRIOL: See VITRIOL, BLUE.

BOHEMIAN BOLE: A pale variegated BOLUS that effervesces slightly with acids.

BOLETUS: See AGARICUS.

BOLUS: "Boles [or Boli] are very viscid clayey earths, less coherent and more friable than clay strictly so called. They are soft and unctuous to the touch, adhere to the tongue and by degrees melt in the mouth, impressing a slight sense of astringency." Astringent, diaphoretic, and alexipharmic. However, the word was sometimes applied to a stiffened soft paste that could be shaped into a pill, and usually contained many ingredients. [15]

BONESET: See EUPATORIUM PERFOLIATUM.

BONTIUS, WATER PILL OF: Made of Socotrine ALOES

and SCAMMONIUM, it was named for 17th–century Dutch physician Jacobus Bontius. Diuretic, cathartic, and deobstruent.

BORACIS, SAL ACIDUM: Same as BORAX.

BORAGE: See BORRAGO.

BORAX: Sodium borate. Sedative, anodyne, refrigerant, febrifuge, antispasmodic, astringent, diuretic, emmenagogue, and emollient. [2,15,23,29]

BORRAGO: Borage, *Borrago officinalis*. Tonic, aperient, and diaphoretic.

BOTRYS: Leaves and seed of Jerusalem oak, *Chenopodium botrys*, var. *anthelminthicum*. An anthelminthic especially suitable for children; carminative, pectoral, and emmenagogue. [2,15,23,29,30] Contains an oil which is effective against hookworms.

BOUGIE: A thin flexible tool for dilating passages of the body, especially the urethra. Made of various materials, including steel and other metals; a soft pliable version was made with CERA FLAVA, SPERMACETI, and CERUSSA ACETATA (the concentration of the latter was increased if more irritation of the passage was desired). Named for the Algerian town from which a suitable wax was exported to France. [15]

BOWMAN'S ROOT: See GILLENIA.

BOX: See BUXUS.

BOXWOOD: Same as CORNUS FLORIDA.

BRASSICA: Cabbage (*Brassica oleracea*), cauliflower (*B. oleracea botrytis*), etc., including sauerkraut. Modestly cathartic and emollient. Sauerkraut was thought to be antiscorbutic, and cabbage leaves were sometimes used to promote continued blistering after application of CANTHARIS. [15] Also see NAPUS and SINAPI.

BRASSICA MARINA: Leaves of sea colewort, Scots scurvygrass, or soldanella, *Convolvulus soldanella*. A strong cathartic. [15]

BRAZIL WOOD: *Caesalpinia echinata*, said to be one source of SANGUIS DRACONIS.

BREAD CRUMBS: See MICA PANIO.

BRICKS, OIL OF: See BRITISH OIL.

BRIMSTONE: Same as SULPHUR.

BRITANNICA, HERBA: See HYDROLAPATHUM.

BRITISH OIL: Originally, a liquid obtained by heating the powder made from bricks that had been soaked in oil or in

OL ROSMARINUS. Later, a PETROLEUM liniment also called "Oil of Bricks" that was patented in 1742 by Michael and Thomas Betton as an antirheumatic and antiscorbutic. The patent was vacated in 1745 when Edmund Darby & Co. proved that they had been manufacturing the same remedy for over a century, but the Bettons' product continued to dominate the market. Later versions were made with OL TEREBINTHA or OL LINI. A panacea. [14]

BROMINE: Discovered by French pharmacist Antoine-Jerôme Balard in 1826. Because of its resemblance to IODINE, it was tried as a medicine and found to stimulate the lymphatic system, and to promote absorption, especially of cutaneous ulcers. [29] Bromides were introduced for the treatment of epilepsy in the 1850s.

BROOKLIME: See BECCABUNGA.

BROOM: See GENISTA and SCOPARIUS; also see RUSCUS.

BRUGNATELLI'S VERMIFUGE POWDER: Tin sulfide.

BRUISEWORT: See SAPONARIA.

BRYONIA: Roots of white bryony, *Bryonia creticum*, subsp. *dioica*, a gourd. Cathartic, diuretic, and an external discutient. [2,15] Contains a drastic cathartic material that can also paralyze the central nervous system.

BUBON GALBANUM: Same as GALBANUM.

BUBULUM, OLEUM: Neat's-foot oil, expressed from bovine feet and shinbones.

BUCHU (or BUCKU): Leaves of buchu, *Barosma betulina*, *B. crenulata*, and/or *B. serratifolia*. Introduced to English medicine from South Africa in 1821. Diuretic and diaphoretic. [29]

BUCK-BEAN: See TRIFOLIUM PALUDOSUM.

BUCKTHORN: See RHAMNUS CATHARTICUS.

BUGBANE: Same as CIMIFUGA.

BUGLEWEED: See LYCOPUS.

BUGLOSSUM: Root and leaves of bugloss, *Anchusa officinalis*, a member of the BORRAGO family. A weak refrigerant. [15]

BURDOCK: See BARDANA.

BURNET SAXIFRAGE: See PIMPINELLA.

BURSA PASTORIS: Leaves of shepherd's purse, *Capsella bursa-pastoris*. A hot astringent or styptic, but not very potent.

BUTCHER'S BROOM: See RUSCUS.

BUTTERBUR: See PETASITIS.
BUTTERCUP: See RANUNCULUS.
BUTTERFLY WEED: See ASCLEPIAS DECUMBENS.
BUTTERNUT: See JUGLANS CINEREA.
BUTTER OF ANTIMONY: Same as ANTIMONIUM MURIATUM.
BUTTER OF LEAD: Lead chloride.
BUTTER OF ZINC: See ZINCI, BUTYRUM.
BUTYRUM: Butter, but not always a dairy product; see, e.g., BUTTER OF ANTIMONY or COCOS BUTYRACEA.
BUXUS: Leaves of box, *Buxus sempervirens*. Cathartic; sometimes said to be diaphoretic. [15]

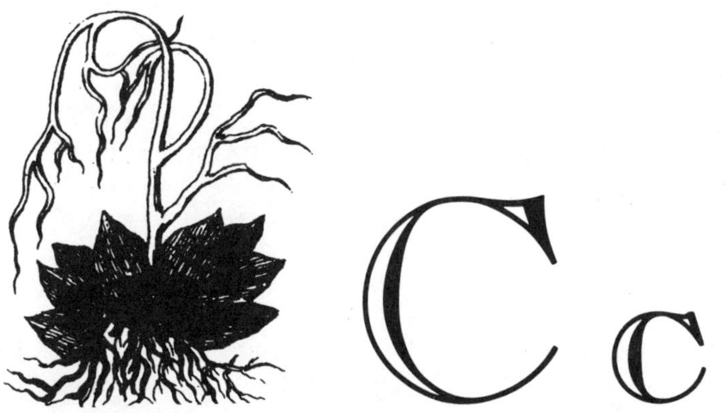

Contrayerva

CABBAGE: See BRASSICA.
CABBAGE TREE: See GEOFFROEA.
CACAO or CACOA: Chocolate nuts, from *Theobroma cacoa*. Although chocolate was known as a drink to the Spanish returning from South America, its medical properties (as a stomachic and antidysenteric) began to emerge only after about 1640. Cocoa butter was introduced to medicine in Germany in the 1730s. Nutritious for patients with consumption. [15] Theobromine was isolated from the seeds in 1842 by Alexander Woskressensky of St. Petersburg.
CACHECTICUS, PULVIS: "Cachectic powder," made with FERRUM, CINNAMOMUM, and SACCHARUM. Restorative.
CAJEPUT: Oil of *Melaleuca leucadendron*. Introduced from the East Indies to the Netherlands in 1727. Used externally as a warm stimulant, antispasmodic, and diaphoretic, for, e.g., toothache, painful joints, and internally "as a very powerful remedy against tympanitic affections." [15,23,30]

CALAMINE: Zinc silicate. Used in skin ointments. [23]

CALAMUS[AROMATICUS]: Roots of sweet flag, *Acorus calamus*. Carminative and stomachic. [15,23,29]

CALCAREO-PHOSPHORATED ANTIMONY: Same as PULVIS ANTIMONIALIS.

CALCII CHLORIDUM: Same as MURIAS CALCIS.

CALCINED ANTIMONY: Same as ANTIMONIUM CALCINATUM.

CALCINED MAGNESIA: Same as MAGNESIA USTA.

CALCINED VITRIOL: Same as FERRUM VITRIOLATUM EXSICCATUM.

CALCIS, AQUA: "Lime water," usually made by dissolving QUICKLIME in water. Commonly used as an astringent with diuretic, diaphoretic, lithontriptic, anthelminthic, and antacid properties. [1,2,15,23]

CALCIS, LINIMENTUM AQUAE: Equal parts of AQUA CALCIS and OL LINUM or OL OLIVA. Applied topically for skin inflammations. [1]

CALENDULA: Flower of the pot marigold, *Calendula* spp., or the garden marigold, *Tagetes* spp. Aperient, alexipharmic, diaphoretic, and emmenagogue, and for small pox. [15]

CALIB., CALYB.: Abbreviations for CHALYBEATE and CHALYBIS.

CAL[L]ICO TREE: See KALMIA LATIFOLIA.

CALOMEL: Mercurous chloride, HgCl, the most widely used of all mercurial drugs from at least 1595. Cathartic, diuretic, emetic, sialagogue, alterative, expectorant, anthelminthic, and antivenereal. [1,2,23,30] Also see HYDRARGYRUS. Calomel may be derived from the Greek for "beautiful black," denoting the source from which the white medicine was prepared. Its mercury ions inhibit the absorption of water and other material from the intestinal lumen.

CALUMBA: Same as COLUMBA.

CALX [VIVA]: Same as QUICKLIME.

CALX CHLORINATA: Calcium hypochlorite, bleaching powder, invented in 1798 by Scottish chemist Smithson Tennant of Glasgow; in 1774 chlorine gas had been discovered, and credited with antiseptic properties, by Swedish chemist Karl Wilhelm Scheele. Used externally as a desiccant and disinfectant, especially for public health purposes, and internally as a tonic and astringent. [29]

CALX HYDRARGYRI ALBA: A precipitate formed by

CALOMEL, SAL AMMONIACUS, and LYE. Used in ointments. [15]

CALYB.: See CALIB.

CAMEL'S HAY: A grass from northern India, *Andropogon schoenanthus*, that yields an aromatic oil called geranium oil. See CALIB.

CAMPECHE: Same as HAEMATOXYLUM.

CAMPHIRE: Same as CAMPHOR.

CAMPHOR: Extract from *Cinnamomum camphora*. Administered both internally and externally, usually in compounded preparations; narcotic (although OPIUM is an antidote), analgesic, anti-inflammatory, diaphoretic, diuretic, tonic, antispasmodic, soporific, antirheumatic, and discutient. Its side effects include vertigo, delirium, and convulsions. [1,15,23,29,30] Camphor is still used in many liniments, but when taken by mouth is hazardous [see Robert Kopelman, Sanford Miller, Raymond Kelly, and Irving Sunshine, "Camphor Intoxication Treated by Resin Hemoperfusion," *Journal of the American Medical Association 241* (1979), 727-728].

CAMPHORATED SPIRIT OF WINE: A liniment made of CAMPHOR in SPIRIT OF WINE.

CANADENSE, BALSAMUM: Volatile oil of Canada balsam, *Abies balsamea*. Tonic, cathartic, and diuretic. [2,15] Also applied to the skin as a topical stimulant. [23]

CANCER ASTACUS: See CANCRORUM LAPILLI.

CANCER, CHELAE: "Crab claws," the black tips of the claws of the common crab, *Cancer pagurus*. Absorbent, antacid, and antidiarrheal.

CANCER PAGURUS: See CANCER, CHELAE.

CANCRORUM LAPILLI: "Little crab stones," white spherical concretions of calcium carbonate found in the gut of the crayfish, *Astacus fluviatilis*; imported from Russia, but often counterfeited with pipe clay. Absorbent antacid, corroborant, and antidiarrheal.

CANCRORUM, OCULI: "Crabs' eyes," a misnomer for CANCRORUM LAPILLI.

CANCRUM EXULCERATUM, UNGUENTUM AD: "Ointment for an ulcerated cancer," made with OL RICINI, WHITE LEAD, and HYDRARGYRUS PRAECIPITATUS. Corrosive. [15]

CANELLA: Literally, "cinnamon." Aromatic inner bark of

Canella alba. Brought to Europe about 1600 from West Indies. Stomachic and gentle tonic. [2,15,29]

CANNA: 1) Starch made from cane, *Canna montana*. 2) Same as MARANTA ARUDINACEA.

CANNABIS: Seed of hemp—marijuana—*Cannabis sativa*. Although known since antiquity, cannabis was reintroduced to European medicine in 1809 by French physicians who had been to Egypt with Napoleon, and again by British army surgeon (and chemist) W. B. O'Shaughnessy, in Calcutta, in 1838. Antitussive; astringent; antaphrodisiac; analgesic and anticonvulsant. [15]

CANTHARIDIS, EMPLASTRUM or UNGUENTUM: Mixture of powdered CANTHARIS (q.v.), CERATE, AXUNGUENTUM PORCINUM, RESINA, and water, applied as a dressing to CANTHARIS-induced blisters to keep them running for up to five days; another was made by melting 24 oz. of adhesive plaster with two oz. of VENICE TURPENTINE, and then stirring in six oz. of finely powdered CANTHARIS beetles. [12] Also used, after dilution, in a friction, or dressing, with CAMPHOR dissolved in WINE, applied locally to stimulate paralyzed muscles. [1] Used as late as 1960 for the same purposes. Also see SINAPI.

CANTHARIDIS, TINCTURA: Dilute alcohol solution of CANTHARIS, q.v. Administered by mouth, after further dilution, as a diuretic, especially for diabetes. [1,15,23]

CANTHARIS, or CANTHARIDES: Powdered "Spanish flies," *Lytta* (formerly *Cantharis*) *vesicatoria*. Usually applied externally as an Epispastic or blistering plaster (i.e., as EMPLASTRUM CANTHARIDIS), it first operates as a general stimulant, to "artificially" remove fluid directly from the body into the blister fluid, and indirectly into urine or phlegm, and then to "relieve torpor" by diverting "the impetus of the blood from the part affected to the part of application." The blister sometimes acts as an antispasmodic or "counter-irritant" that reflexly reduces irritability, especially of the blood vessels, thereby altering the circulation in patients with severe fevers, but sometimes to stimulate the vascular and nervous tissues in adjacent anatomical areas by "counter-irritation." [1,2,15,20,23,29,30] Some American physicians said that an extract of the potato fly, which they called Lytta Vittata, probably the potato bug or beetle, *Leptinotarsa decemlineata*, was equally effective as a blister and diuretic. [23, pp. 262-264]

An 1849 method for applying a cantharis plaster recommended that "It should be spread on soft leather, though linen or even paper will [suffice]. An elegant mode of preparing it for use is to spread a piece of leather, of a proper size, first with adhesive plaster, and afterwards with the [cantharis] cerate, leaving a margin of the [leather] uncovered, in order that it may adhere to the skin. . . Upon the application of the plaster, the skin should be moistened with warm vinegar or other liquid; and a good rule is to cover the surface of the plaster closely with very thin gauze or unsized paper, which prevents any of the cerate from adhering to the cuticle [i.e., the epidermis]. . . In the case of adults, when the full action of the flies is desired, and the object is to produce a permanent effect, the application should be continued for twelve hours, and on the scalp for twenty-four hours. In very delicate persons, however, . . or when the object is merely to produce a blister to be healed as quickly as possible, the plaster should remain no longer than is necessary for the production of full redness of the skin, which generally occurs in five or six hours. . . It should then be removed, and followed by a bread and milk poultice, or some other emollient dressing, under which the cuticle rises, and a full blister is usually produced. . . [T]he blister will very quickly heal after the discharge of the serum. . . After the blister has been formed, it should be opened at the most depending parts, and, the cuticle being allowed to remain, should be dressed with simple cerate; but, if it be desirable to maintain the discharge for a short time, resin cerate should be used, and the cuticle removed, if it can be done without inconvenience. When it is desirable that the blistered surface should heal as soon as possible, . . . Dr. Maclagan recommends a dressing of cotton wadding; an emollient poultice being first applied for two hours after the removal of the blistering cerate, the cuticle then cut, and the surface afterwards covered with the cotton, with its raw surface next the skin. Should the dressing become soaked with the serous discharge, so much of the cotton may be removed as can be done without disturbing the cuticle, and a new batch applied. The cotton may be allowed to remain until the old cuticle spontaneously separates." [30, pp. 886-887]

For the drug's internally administered form, see TINCTURA CANTHARIDIS. When taken undiluted by mouth, cantharis produced severe dysuria, abdominal pain, hematuria, bloody stools, thirst, fetid breath, "madness," and death (the latter was presumably caused by the cardiac arrhythmia produced by the drug's active principle, cantharidin). Its ability to irritate the lower urinary tract and thereby produce a prolonged erection (following either topical or internal administration) gave rise to the aphrodisiacal mythology of Spanish fly. The toxicity of the active ingredient of extracts of the Spanish fly (actually, a beetle that is indigenous to the eastern Mediterranean littoral), cantharidin (extracted by French chemist Pierre-Jean Robiquet in 1810), was explored recently in: Simon W. Rabkin, Janet M. Friesen, John A.J. Ferris, and Henry Y.M. Fung, "A Model of Cardiac Arrhythmias and Sudden Death: Cantharidin-induced Toxic Cardiomyopathy," *Journal of Pharmacology and Experimental Therapeutics, 210* (1979), 43-50. Also see Peter V. Taberner, *Aphrodisiacs: The Science and the Myth* (Philadelphia: University of Pennsylvania Press, 1985), pp. 102-111. The toxicity of cantharis pills was the subject of a malpractice case reported by Harold J. Cook in *The Decline of the Old Medical Regime in Stuart London* (Ithaca, N.Y.: Cornell University Press, 1986), pp. 240-242. Cantharidin preparations are still available for the removal of benign skin growths such as warts.

CANTHIANUS, PULVIS: "Powder of Kent;" same as CANCER LAPILLI.

CAPERS: See CAPPARIS.

CAPIVI: Same as COPAIVA.

CAPPARIS: Root bark and buds of caper bush, *Capparis spinosa*. Aperient, diuretic, and deobstruent; pickled buds stimulate the appetite. [15]

CAPSELLA: See BURSA PASTORIS.

CAPSICUM [ANNUUM]: Same as PIPER INDICUM.

CAPUCHINS, POWDER OF: "Capuchin [Monks'] Powder;" made of STAPHISAGRIA, NICOTIANA, and SABADILLA.

CAPUT MORTUUM: "Dead head;" usually potassium chloride precipitated during distillation of SAL AMMONIAC, but occasionally same as FERRI RUBIGO. Antihysteric and febrifuge; digestive (def. no. 2). [15]

CARAWAY: See CARUM.

CARBO LIGNI: Same as PULVIS CARBONAS LIGNI.

CARBONAS AMMONIAE, or AQUA CARBONAS AMMONIAE: Same as AMMONIAE PRAEPARATA. [23]

CARBONAS BARYTES: Barium carbonate, or witherite (named for Dr. William Withering, who discovered this rare mineral in 1783; see DIGITALIS). Poisonous; used only in manufacture of MURIAS BARYTAE.

CARBONAS CALCIS PRAEPARATUS: Same chemical composition as CRETA.

CARBONAS CALCIS, SAL: Calcium carbonate. Antacid. [1,2] Applied topically to burns.

CARBONAS FERRI [PRAECIPITATUS]: Ferrous carbonate, but probably really FERRI RUBIGO. Tonic. [23]

CARBONAS LIGNI, PULVIS: Powdered charcoal. Absorbent and antiseptic. [1,15,23,29,30] Also see CHARCOAL AND KALI SULPHURATUM.

CARBONAS MAGNESIAE: Same as MAGNESIA ALBA.

CARBONAS PLUMBI: Same as WHITE LEAD.

CARBONAS POTASSAE [IMPURUS]: Same as LIXIVA.

CARBONAS POTASSAE PURISSIMUS: Same as SAL TARTARI.

CARBONAS SODAE: Sodium carbonate, or purified BARILLA. Antacid, deobstruent, lithontriptic, attenuant, diaphoretic, diuretic, and tonic. [23,29]

CARBONAS ZINCI: Zinc carbonate. Used in collyria. [23]

CARBONAS ZINCI IMPURUS PRAEPARATUS: Same as CALAMINE.

CARBONATIS AMMONIAE, AQUA: Same as AQUA AMMONIAE.

CARBONICI, AQUA ACIDI: Soda, or carbonated, water. Febrifuge, antiemetic, and diuretic.

CARBONICUM, ACIDUM: Carbonic acid, carbon dioxide, or FIXED AIR.

CARDAMINE: Flowers of ladies' smock, or cuckoo-flower, *Cardamine pratensis*. Diuretic, antispasmodic, and occasionally diaphoretic. [15,29]

CARDAMOM, LESSER: See CARDAMOMUM MINUS.

CARDAMOMUM MINUS: Seeds of lesser cardamom, *Eletteria cardamomum*. Aromatic, carminative, and diaphoretic. [15]

Cardiac: A drug used to treat dyspepsia or heartburn, because the upper part of the stomach is called the cardia.

CARDIACA, AQUA: "Cardiac water," a solution of CIN-

NAMOMUM, CARDAMOMUM MINUS, ZINGIBER, and CORTEX AURANTIUM (also see AROMATIC ELECTUARY, def. no. 1). Digestive, def. no. 1. [1]

CARDIACA, CONFECTIO: Same as def. no. 2 for AROMATIC ELECTUARY.

CARDIAC DROPS: Same as AQUA CARDIACA.

CARDIALGIA, TABELLA: Digestive (def. no. 1) lozenges.

CARDUUS BENEDICTUS: Blessed thistle, *Centaurea benedicta*. Tonic, diaphoretic, and emetic, as dose increases. [15,23,29]

CARICA: Dried fig, *Ficus carica*. Sweet emollient laxative; promotes suppuration of superficial wounds and under cataplasms. [15,23,29]

CARLINA: Root of carline thistle, *Carlina vulgaris*, or other spp. Diaphoretic, alexipharmic, and occasionally emetic. [15]

CARMELITANA, AQUA: "Carmelite water," a panacea first made at a Carmelite monastery in Paris in 1611, patented in 1709 and again in 1780, and sold as late as 1866, although the formula had been slightly modified by then. Made of MELISSA, CORTEX LIMONI, NUTMEG, CORIANDRUM, CARYOPHYLLUS AROMATICUS, CINNAMOMUM, and alcohol. [13,15]

Carminative: A drug that facilitates expulsion of gas from the intestines; most often prescribed for dyspepsia.

CAROLINA PINKROOT: See SPIGELIA.

CAROTA: Seed of DAUCUS SYLVESTRIS.

CARPOBALSAMUM: Fruit of *Commiphora opobalsamum*. Used in THERIAC and other complex mixtures. [15] Also see BALM OF GILEAD.

CARRAGEEN: Same as CHONDRUS.

CARROT, CANDY: See DAUCUS CRETICUS.

CARROT, DEADLY: See SILPHIUM.

CARROT, WILD: See DAUCUS SYLVESTRIS.

CARTHAMUS: Seeds of bastard saffron thistle, safflower, or dyer's saffron, *Carthamus tinctorius*. Diaphoretic and cathartic. [15,29,30]

CARTHUSIANUS, PULVIS: "Carthusian [Monks'] powder;" same as KERMES MINERALE.

CARUM, CARUON, or CARVI: Seeds of caraway, *Carum carvi*. Stomachic, carminative, and diuretic. [15,23,29]

CARYOCOSTINUM, ELECTUARIUM: An early formulation of ELECTUARIUM SCAMMONII.

CARYOPHYLLATA: Root of water avens, or herb bennet,

Geum urbanum (and other *Geum* spp.) Tonic, stomachic, astringent, and antiseptic. [15, 23,29,30] Also see GEUM RIVALE.

CARYOPHYLLUM RUBRUM: Flowers of July-flowers, *Dianthus caryophyllus*. Cardiac and alexipharmic, but used chiefly only for flavoring. [15]

CARYOPHYLLUS AROMATICUS: Cloves, the dried buds of *Eugenia aromatica*. Hot stimulating aromatic; also, somewhat styptic. [15,23,29]

CASCARILLA: Bark of *Croton eleutheria* (and other spp.). Brought to England from East Indies soon after 1630, and known to medicine by 1693. It was named "cascarilla," meaning "little bark," because it resembled CINCHONA, usually called simply "Bark." Astringent tonic; sometimes used as a substitute for CINCHONA. [2,15,23,29,30]

CASHUB: Same as LIXIVA.

CASSIAE, ELECTUARIUM: Made with CASSIA, MANNA, TAMARINDUS, and syrup of ROSES. Cathartic. [15]

CASSIA FISTULA: Pod of *Cassia fistula* (or *C. marilandica* in the U.S.). A mild cooling cathartic; turns urine green. [1,15,29]

CASSIA LIGNEA: Bark and buds of *Laurus cassia*. Substitute for CINNAMOMUM. [15]

CASSIA SENNA: Same as SENNA.

CASSIUS, PURPLE POWDER OF: A compound of AURUM and STANNUM discovered by 17th–century German physician and chemist Andreas Cassius. Antivenereal, but not well documented. [23]

CASTANEA: Bark of chinquapin tree, *Castanea pumila*. Tonic and astringent; sometimes used as a substitute for CINCHONA. [29,30]

CASTELLI, DIATARTARI OF: See DIATARTARI.

CASTILE, SOAP OF: See SAPO ALBUS.

CASTOR[EUM]: A fatty material from the glands lying between the anus and external genitalia of the Russian beaver, *Castor fiber*; a less potent material was found in American beavers, *C. americanus*. Nerve tonic, antiemetic, antispasmodic, antihysteric, and emmenagogue. [15,23,29]

CASTOREI, TINCTURA: Alcohol extract of CASTOREUM and ASAFOETIDA. A potent antihysteric. [15]

CASTOR FIBER: Same as CASTOREUM.

CASTOR OIL: Same as OL RICINI.

CASUMUNAR: A tuberous root from an unknown plant of the East Indies. Antihysteric, stomachic, and carminative. [15]

Catagmatica: External remedies for bone fractures.

Cataplasm: A watery (not oily) poultice.

Catapotia: Pills.

CATARIA: Same as NEPETA.

CATECHU: 1) Extract of wood of *Areca catechu*. It first entered European markets from India and Burma via Japan (hence it was sometimes called Terra Japonica) in the 1670s. Astringent, tonic; expectorant; used in several compound drugs, especially antidiarrheals. [1,2,15,23,29] The seed contains the cholinergic alkaloid arecoline. 2) Far less often, extract of *Uncaria gambir*. Brought from East Indies to the Netherlands in 1780. Same properties as those for def. no. 1 above.

CATECHU, ELECTUARIUM: Made with CATECHU, OPIUM, GUM KINO, CINNAMOMUM, NUTMEG, and syrup of ROSES. A relatively weak opiate resembling DIASCORDIUM. [15]

CATECHU, INFUSUM: Infusion made with CATECHU, CINNAMOMUM, and simple syrup. Antidiarrheal but also cathartic. [1]

Cathaeritica: Wound ointments.

Cathartic: A medicine that augments the natural peristaltic flow of intestinal contents to excite defecation, or to increase fluid secretion from the intestinal lining ("hydragogue cathartics"); some also act on neighboring organs to increase bile flow (as cholagogues) and gastric emptying. Used to treat constipation, but far more often as antiphlogistic therapy in, e.g., colic, dysentery, fevers, dyspepsia, hypochondriasis, amenorrhea, jaundice, dropsy, apoplexy, coma, mania, headache, and rheumatism.

CATHARTIC DULCIS: "Gentle cathartic." Same as CALOMEL.

CATHARTICUS AMARUS, SAL: "Bitter cathartic salt," MAGNESIA VITRIOLATA.

CATHARTICUS, SAL: "Cathartic salt," a frequent synonym for VITRIOLATED SODA, but other cathartics may also be meant.

Catholicon: A panacea; originally, an electuary that purged all the humors.

CATNIP: See NEPETA.

Catoterica: Cathartics that empty the kidneys, bladder, and liver.

Caustic: An escharotic (q.v.) drug; if appropriately diluted, many caustics were cathartic and anthelminthic when ingested, and lithontriptic when instilled directly into the bladder.

CAUSTIC ALKALINE LIXIVA: Same as LYE.

CAUSTIC LEY: Same as AQUA POTASSAE.

CAUSTIQUE PERPETUEL: "Permanent caustic," ARGENTUM NITRATUM.

CAYENNE PEPPER: See PIPER INDICUM.

CELANDINE: See CHELIDONIUM MAJUS and MINUS.

CELERY, WILD: See APIUM.

CENTAUREA BENEDICTA: Same as CARDUUS BENEDICTA.

CENTAURIUM MAJOR: Root of greater centaury, either of two members of the GENTIAN family, *Centaureum umbellatum* or *Chlora perfoliata*. Tonic astringent, aperient, and vulnerary. [15]

CENTAURIUM MINUS: Tops of lesser centaury, *Centaureum ramoissimum* or *C. umbellatum*. Aperient. [15,23]

CENTAURY, AMERICAN: 1) Flowers of American knapweed, *Centaurea americana*. Used as a substitute for CENTAURIUM MAJOR. [29] 2) Same as SABBATIA.

CEPA: Onion, *Allium cepa*. Appetite stimulant; diuretic, diaphoretic, and expectorant; used in discutient cataplasms to promote suppuration. [15,29] Also see GARLIC.

Cephalic: A remedy for disorders of the head (e.g., headache, coma, epilepsy, and palsy).

CEPHALICUM, EMPLASTRUM: Same as EMPLASTRUM PICIS BURGUNDICAE COMPOSITUM.

CERA ALBA: White beeswax, i.e., sun-bleached CERA FLAVA. Used to make plasters, unguents, etc.; sometimes given internally as an intestinal emollient. [15]

CERAE COMPOSITUM, EMPLASTRUM: Plaster made of CERA FLAVA, OVIS, and OL TEREBINTHA, often applied as a dressing after blistering with CANTHARIS.

CERA FLAVA: Yellow beeswax. Uses same as for CERA ALBA.

CERASI, AQUA: Made by bruising CERASUS berries and seeds in water. A mild cathartic, it had been abandoned by the 1790s because of its "opium-like" toxicity [15], perhaps caused by the hydrocyanic acid released from the broken seeds. See PRUNUS LAUROCERASUS.

CERASUS: Leaves, fruit, and gum of the wild sour (or black) cherry, *Prunus cerasus*, and related spp. Refrigerant; aperient. [15] Tonic, slightly narcotic, anthelminthic, and antiseptic. [23]

Cerate: An external application with a consistency between those of plasters and unguents (i.e., with more wax.)

CERATE: Beeswax.

CERATE, LINIMENT: CALAMINE in CERATE or oils. Astringent emollient. [2]

Ceratomalagmata: Cerates.

CEREFOLIUM: Chervil, *Anthriscus cerefolium*. Gentle aperient; diuretic. [15]

Cerevisiae: Medicines made by fermentation with malt, i.e., medicinal beers.

CEREVISIAE FERMENTUM: Yeast. Tonic and antiseptic; sometimes used in cataplasms. [29]

CERONEUM: A plaster made with CERA ALBA (or CERA FLAVA) and CROCUS.

CERRALINA: Same as GALLA.

CERUSSA or CERUSSE: 1) Same as CERUSSA ACETATA. 2) Less often, WHITE LEAD. 3) Now applied to lead carbonate, with the approximate formula $(PbCO_3)_2 \cdot Pb(OH)_2$.

CERUSSA ACETATA: Lead acetate. Used as a cooling collyrium, or internally as a styptic astringent, an anti-diaphoretic, or an anti-inflammatory sedative. An oral overdose produces colic, constipation, cramps, tremors, and nerve weakness; also see PLUMBUM. [1,2,15,23,29]

CERUSSA ACETATAE, UNGUENTUM: Ointment made with CERUSSA ACETATA and UNGUENTUM SIMPLEX. A cooling and desiccating skin ointment. [1]

CERUSSA ANTIMONII: Antimony nitrate. Cathartic. [15]

CERVUS ELAPHUS: Same as HARTSHORN.

CETACEUM: Same as SPERMACETI.

CETRARIA: Same as LICHEN ISLANDICUS.

CEVADILLA: See SABADILLA.

Chalastica: Emollients.

CHALK: See CRETA.

CHALYBEATE: 1) Iron tartrates (actually, probably FERRI RUBIGO) in wine. Astringent. 2) Usually means any medicine made with FERRUM or one of its salts; also used alone to treat chlorosis. [2] A typical chalybeate pill would "invigorate impoverished blood, strengthen the stomach, assist digestion, open obstructions, and promote menstrual discharge." [12]

CHALYBEATUM, VINUM: Same as VINUM FERRI.

CHALYBIS, [SAL]: Same as FERRUM VITRIOLATUM.

CHAMAEDRYS: Germander, mints of genus *Teucrium*. Diaphoretic, diuretic, emmenagogue, and stomachic. [15]

CHAMAEMELUM: Dried powdered flowers of chamomile, sometimes called Roman chamomile, *Anthemis nobilis*. Tonic, diaphoretic, antiseptic, antispasmodic, antihysteric, carminative, digestive, and aperient; vermifuge; emollient and discutient. [2,15,23,29]

CHAMAEPITHYS: European groundpine, *Ajuga chamaepithys*. Aperient; also, vulnerary and antirheumatic. [15]

CHAMOMILE: See CHAMAEMELUM and MATRICARIA.

CHAMOMILE, WILD: See COTULA FOETIDA.

CHARCOAL: Same as PULVIS CARBONAS LIGNI.

CHARCOAL AND KALI SULPHURATUM: About 1790 Dr. Thomas Garnett of Harrogate, England, devised this mixture of charcoal and potassium sulfate for the treatment of phthisis (consumption), based on the following rationale: according to Dr. Thomas Beddoes, phthisis was caused by, or associated with, hyperoxygenation of the blood; therefore, Garnett reasoned, after the drug mixture enters the blood from the intestines, "the Chyle is impregnated with the sulphurated hydrogenous Gas, which unites with the Oxygen of the Blood & forms Water," thereby removing the excess oxygen from the blood. [1]

CHARTREUX, POUDRE DE: "Powder of Chartreux," KERMES MINERALE.

CHECKERBERRY: See GAULTHERIA.

CHELAE CANCER: See CANCER, CHELAE.

CHELARUM CANCRI COMPOSITUS, PULVIS: "Compound powder of crab claws," a mixture of CANCER LAPILLI, CRETA, and CORALLIUM RUBRUM. [15]

CHELIDONIUM MAJUS: Leaves and root of celandine, *Chelidonium majus*. Aperient, diuretic, and diaphoretic, especially in jaundice, because the root is yellow. Used for eye disorders in folk medicine, although it is acrid, and for warts. [15]

CHELIDONIUM MINUS: Root of pilewort, or lesser celandine, *Ficaria verna*. Used in folk medicine for piles because parts of the roots resemble hemorrhoids. [15]

CHELSEA PENSIONER: An 18th-century antirheumatic electuary associated with the Chelsea Hospital founded by Charles II for aged or disabled soldiers. Its formula varied, but usually included GUIAC, RHEI, and SULPHUR.

CHENOPODIUM [ANTHELMINTICUM]: Same as BOTRYS.

CHENOPODIUM VULVARIA: See ATRIPLEX FOETIDA.

CHERMES: Same as KERMES.

CHERRY: See CERASUS and PRUNUS VIRGINIANUS.

CHERVIL: See CEREFOLIUM.

CHESTNUT, HORSE: See HIPPOCASTANUM.

CHESTNUT, WATER: See WATER CALTROP.

CHICORY: See CICHOREUM.

CHIMAPHILA: Leaves of pipsissewa, or prince's pine, *Chimaphila umbellata*. Diuretic, tonic, and astringent. [29]

CHINA: 1) China root, *Smilax china*. Introduced to Europe from the East Indies by the Portuguese in 1525. A diaphoretic and diuretic used for venereal and skin disorders. [15] 2) Same as CINCHONA.

CHINA BERRY: Same as MELIA AZEDARACH.

CHINAE, CORTEX: Dr. Georg Ernest Stahl's term (1708) for CINCHONA.

CHINA, PRIDE OF: Same as MELIA AZEDARACH.

CHINQUAPIN: See CASTANEA.

CHIRETTA: Stems and roots of *Ophelia* (or *Agathotes*) *chirayta*. Introduced from India to England by 1829. Bitter tonic; cholagogue; cathartic. [29]

CHIRONIA CENTAURIUM: Probably same as CENTAURIUM MINUS.

CHLOROFORM: Discovered in 1831 by apothecary Eugène Soubeiran in France, Dr. Justus von Liebig in Germany, and Dr. Samuel Guthrie in the U.S., and named by Jean Baptiste Dumas in 1835. In 1847, Dr. Jacob Bell in England, and French physiologist Marie-Jean-Pierre Flourens, used it to produce anesthesia in animals, and Dr. James Y. Simpson of Edinburgh used it to produce obstetrical anesthesia.

CHOCOLATE: See CACAO.

CHOCOLATE ROOT: See GEUM RIVALE.

Cholagoga: Remedies that purge the bilious humor.

CHONDRODENDRON TOMENTOSUM: See PAREIRA BRAVA.

CHONDRUS: Irish moss, *Chondrus crispus*, an edible North Atlantic seaweed introduced to medicine in 1831. Nutritive and demulcent. [29]

CHRISTMAS ROSE: See HELLEBORUS NIGER.

CHYLISTA: ANTIMONIUM VITRIFICATUM mixed with MASTICHE and SPIRIT OF WINE. Cathartic. [15]

CICERA TARTARI: "Peas of tartar." Pills of TEREBINTHA and CREAM OF TARTAR. Also see MYNSICHT'S CICERA TARTARI.

CICHOREUM: Chicory, or succory, *Chicorium intybus* (or sometimes endive, *C. endivia*). Cathartic, intestinal tonic, stomachic, blood purifier, and refrigerant. [15]

CICUTA: Leaves of modern poison hemlock, *Conium maculatum*. Initially promoted by Dr. Anton Störck of Vienna about 1760. Given internally, in small doses, as a potent (albeit only palliative) tonic narcotic and sedative, or applied externally as a discutient. Poisonous in large doses, its principal manifestation is weakness and eventual muscle paralysis, but it also produces vertigo, dim vision, difficult speech, nausea, anxiety, tremors, mydriasis, and delirium, stupor, terminal convulsions, and death by respiratory muscle paralysis. [1,23,29,30] The active alkaloid, coniine (or conine), which comprises about 0.8% of the leaf, was isolated by Gieseke in 1827. N.B.: The modern water hemlock, or cowbane, is *Cicuta maculata*; although it can produce similar symptoms, by contrast it causes tonic-clonic convulsions. Also see OENANTHE, which can produce a similar syndrome.

CIMIFUGA: Root of black snakeroot, black cohosh, or bugbane, *Cimifuga racemosa*. Mild tonic, diaphoretic, diuretic, expectorant, and emmenagogue; sedative. [29,30]

CINARA: Juice and leaves of artichoke, *Cynara scolamus*. Diuretic. [15]

CINCHONA [OFFICINALIS]: Usually the powdered bark called pale or crown bark, from *Cinchona officinalis*, was meant. Sometimes "Cinchona Flavus" (yellow bark) or "Cinchona Rubra" (red bark) was specified. However, although it is commonly believed that these pigmented barks may have come from *C. calisaya* and *C. succirubra*, respectively, the technical and vernacular nomenclatures of *Cinchona* species are not at all clear [29, pp. 212-234]. The barks of other species may be yellow and red as well, so that it is not possible to ascertain precisely which species were used therapeutically merely by the reported or prescribed colors of the bark. At least both *C. calisaya* and *C. succirubra* are known to have been found in Peru, the chief source of the drug, by the late 18th century. Modern laboratory analyses show that the concentration of quinine varies not only in the bark from species to species but also in different parts of one tree, from year to year, and from one region to another. This means that, while the pale barks were prescribed more often than the colored varieties and were more often therapeutically effective, information about the color of a given preparation cannot help identify it by its species. [For the botanical problems involved, see: Leo Suppan, "Three Centuries of Cinchona," in *Proceedings of the Celebration of the Three Hundredth Anniversary ofthe First Recognized Use of Cinchona*, 31 October-1 November 1930 (St. Louis: Missouri Botanical Garden, 1930), pp. 29-138.]

After its introduction to European medicine in the 1630s, and to England about 1655, cinchona was widely used as a tonic, as an astringent, and as an antiseptic, especially for patients with intermittent fevers (i.e., the malarias), for dyspepsia (i.e., impaired digestion), and for spasmodic symptoms of chest disease, such as cough. It was also prescribed for most patients who had been debilitated by continued fevers, and, for venereal disease patients, in a gargle made with CONSERVE OF ROSES, to counteract the side effects of therapeutic mercury in the oral cavity. Cinchona's side effects included vomiting (minimized by administering it in red wine), diarrhea (prevented by the concomitant administration of OPIUM), tachycardia, tinnitus, and partial deafness. [15,23,29,30]

Cinchona was not regarded as a "specific" (q.v.) for intermittent or other fevers. Dr. William Cullen of Edinburgh reasoned that, because its effects can be perceived soon after it is ingested but before it can be absorbed into the blood, its tonic powers must be conveyed via nerves from the stomach to the rest of the body. Therefore, he went on, cinchona is not appropriate therapy for patients with phlogistic (inflammatory) disorders, because they would only worsen under such a stimulating influence, but it would be appropriate for patients with debility induced by continued fevers, after remissions of phlogistic disorders have begun, or after inflammatory symptoms have been removed. Cinchona's remarkable therapeutic success rate in the intermittent fevers led to its earliest trials in continued fevers. [1,2,46; William Cullen, *First Lines of the Practice of Physic*, new ed., 4 vols. (Edinburgh and London, 1789), I, 245-247]

Although Dr. Andrew Duncan, Sr., of Edinburgh, prepared a precipitate of the active principle in 1803, purified quinine was first prepared by French chemists Pierre-Joseph Pelletier and Joseph-Bienaimée Caventou in 1811. In 1749, Dr. Jean–Baptiste de Senac of Paris corrected a cardiac arrhythmia with cinchona, but not until 1914 was quinidine, an isomer of quinine, found to be regularly effective in controlling such arrhythmias, by Dr. Karl Friedrich Wenckebach of Vienna (although it had been isolated in 1848 and named by Louis Pasteur in 1853). Cinchona barks contain about 8% quinine and up to 3% quinidine.

CINCHONAE, TINCTURA: Same as HUXHAM'S TINCTURE.

CINERES CLAVELLATI: Same as LIXIVA.

CINNABAR (or CINNABARIS NATIVA): Red mercuric sulfide, mercury ore. Sialagogue, diaphoretic, and antiepileptic. Side effects include nausea, vomiting, and anxiety. [2,15]

CINNAMOMI COMPOSITA, TINCTURA: Same as TINCTURA AROMATICA.

CINNAMOMUM: Bark of *Cinnamomum zeylanicum* or *C. lourerii*. Tonic, aromatic, stomachic, carminative, and astringent. [2,15,23,29]

CINQUEFOIL: See PENTAPHYLLUM.

CITRICUM, ACIDUM: The sour principle of citrus fruits (but not their antiscorbutic principle). Used chiefly as a flavoring, especially in effervescent waters. Also see LIMON.

CITRINE OINTMENT: A skin unguent said to have been devised in 1596, it first contained limpet shells, quartz, marble, CORALLINA, CERUSSA, and GUM TRAGACANTH in a mixture of animal fats; by the end of the 17th century it was made of CERUSSA ACETATA, AQUA ROSAE, FRANKINCENSE and bark of CITRUS. A collyrium version was made of HYDRARGYRUS NITRATUS in AXUNGUENTUM PORCINUM. [13] In the early 20th century it contained HYDRARGYRUS, ACIDUM NITRICUM, and lard, and was prescribed for many skin diseases.

CITRON: See CITRUS.

CITRULLUS COLOCYNTHIS: See COLOCYNTHIS.

CITRUS: Fruit of the citron, *Citrus medica*. Used as LIMON (q.v.) is. [15]

CITRUS AURANTIUM: Same as AURANTIUM CORTEX.

CITRUS MEDICA: Same as LIMON.

CLARY: See HORMINUM SATIVUM.

CLAVOS PEDUM, EMPLASTRUM AD: "Corn plaster," made with GALBANUM, PIX, DIACHYLON, VERDEGRIS, and SAL AMMONIAC.

CLEMATIS: See FLAMULA JOVIS.

CLOVER: See MELLILOT.

CLOVES: See CARYOPHYLLUS AROMATICUS.

Clyster: A glyster.

COCCIA (or COCHIA), PILULE: The ancient original formulation of PILULE ALOES CUM COLOCYNTHIDE (q.v.), made with ALOES, COLOCYNTHIS, SCAMMONIUM, and ABSINTHUM VULGARE (or CARYOPHYLLUS AROMATICUS). Cathartic. [15,23]

COCCINELLA: Same as COCHINEAL.

COCCULUS: Berries of *Anamirta cocculus*, used in the East Indies to poison fish. Used only for topical treatment of cutaneous eruptions. [29] Its active principle is picrotoxin, a potent convulsant isolated by French pharmacist Pierre François Guillaume Boullay in 1812.

COCCUS: See LACCA.

COCCUS CACTI: Same as COCHINEAL.

COCHIAE MAJOR, PILULE: Same as PILULE COCCIA.

COCHIAE MINOR, PILULE: Same as COCCIA with RHAMNUS CATHARTICUS added. Strong cathartic.

COCHINEAL: Brilliant red dye (now known as carmine red) made from females of a tropical American scale insect, *Dactylopius coccus*. Sometimes recommended as a diaphoretic, cardiac, antitussive, and alexipharmic, but, by the late 18th century, chiefly used only to color several drugs. [2,15,29; Thomas Eisner, Stephen Nowicki, Michael Goetz, and Jerrold Meinwald, "Red Cochineal Dye (Carminic Acid): Its Role in Nature," *Science 208* (1980): 1039-1042]

Cochl[eare]: Spoonful; see Measurement.

COCHLEARIA ARMORACIA: Same as RAPHANUS RUSTICANUS.

COCHLEARIA COMPOSITUS, SUCCUS: Compound

juices of COCHLEARIA HORTENSIS, NASTURTIUM AQUATICUM, and AURANTIUM HISPALENSE, as well as NUTMEG. Antiscorbutic. [15]

COCHLEARIA HORTENSIS: Scurvygrass, *Cochlearia officinalis.* An antiscorbutic diuretic and aperient; also used in gargles for scorbutic gums. [15,23,29]

COCHLEARIA MARINA: Sea scurvygrass, *Cochlearia anglica.* Antiscorbutic. [15]

COCHLEARIA OFFICINALIS: Same as COCHLEARIA HORTENSIS.

COCOA: Same as CACAO, q.v.

COCOS BUTYRACEA: "Cocoa butter," see CACAO; also, sometimes same as PALMA.

COCTUS, SAL: Same as SAL MURIATICUS.

CODEINE: See OPIUM.

COD-LIVER OIL: Oil from liver of cod, *Gadus morhua*, or related species. First used in England in 1785, and recommended by European physicians in the 1820s, but not found in standard compendia until much later. Now known to contain large amounts of vitamins A and D.

COFFEA: Coffee, *Coffea arabica.* Introduced to Europe in the early 17th century. Astringent, antiseptic, and strongly tonic. Used to stimulate digestion and all natural secretions (e.g., to provoke diuresis), to "remove a disposition to sleepiness," and to treat "spasmodic asthma" and severe headache. [15,20,23] In 1820, Friedlieb Ferdinand Runge, of Breslau, isolated caffeine from tea leaves, and a year later French chemist Pierre Jean Robiquet found it in coffee.

COHOSH, BLACK: See CIMIFUGA.

COLCHICUM: Root (actually, the corm) of meadow saffron, *Colchicum autumnale.* Although known since antiquity, it was widely neglected because of its toxicity until Dr. Anton Störck of Vienna and others began to popularize it in the 1760s. Used chiefly as an anodyne narcotic in gout and as a potent but undependable diuretic and diaphoretic in various fevers. Side effects include vomiting, bloody stools, severe abdominal pain, bradycardia, and stupor, as the dose increases. [15,29] The active alkaloid, colchicine, isolated in 1833 by Philipp Lorenz Geiger and Germain Henri Hess of Heidelberg, is still important in the therapy of gout.

COLCOTHAR: Same as FERRI RUBIGO.

COLCOTHAR OF VITRIOL: Same as FERRUM VITRIOLATUM EXSICCATUM.

COLD WATER: Applied over the kidneys to stimulate them to excrete fluid that has accumulated in the body. [1]

Collution: A liquid mouthwash.

Collutory: A medicine with the consistency of honey to be applied to the gums.

Collyrium: A medication (fluid or dry) to be applied topically to the eyes for inflammatory conditions such as ophthalmia.

COLOCYNTHIDIS, EXTRACTUM COMPOSITUM: "Compound extract of colocynth." Made of COLOCYNTHIS, ALOES, SCAMMONIUM, and CARDAMOMUM MINUS. Cathartic. [15]

COLOCYNTHIS: Pulp of fruit of *Citrullus colocynthus*. A potent and violent cathartic that can produce bloody stools; often used in combination with other cathartics to potentiate them, and so that the others will ameliorate the effects of the colocynth. [1,15,23,29,30] Still sometimes used as a cathartic; it irritates the small intestine so as to inhibit the reabsorption of water from the lumen.

COLT'S FOOT: See TUSSILAGO.

COLUMBA (or COLUMBO): Powdered root of *Swertia caroliniensis* (or *Jateorhiza palmata*). Brought to Europe by the Portuguese in the 17th century, it was introduced to medicine in 1671, and promoted in the late 18th century by Dr. Thomas Percival of Manchester and Dr. Hieronymus David Gaub of Heidelberg. Mild tonic, antiseptic, or antiemetic; thought to be astringent in the 18th century, but not in the 19th. [1,2,15,23,29] Its bitter principle, columbine, was isolated in 1832, and berberine (see BERBERIS) was isolated in 1848.

COLUMBA, AMERICAN: Root of *Frasera caroliniensis* (or *F. waltheri*). Same properties as COLUMBA.

COMFREY: See CONSOLIDA.

COMMANDEUR, BAUME DE: Originally a panacea and vulnerary based on FERRUM that was devised about 1680 by Gaspart, lord of Pernes (near Avignon), and a commander in the Knights of Malta. By the late 18th century, it was a liniment much like TINCTURA BENZOINI COMPOSITA.

COMMITISSAE, PULVIS: "Powder of the Countess [of Cinchon]," who was supposed to have introduced it to European medicine in 1640; same as CINCHONA.

COMMON PLASTER: Same as DIACHYLON.

COMMUNIS, EMULSIO: Same as LAC AMYGDALAE.

Composing pill: A sleeping pill. Most included OPIUM.

Confection: An electuary, for practical purposes.

Cong[ius]: Gallon; see Measurement.

CONIUM [MACULATUM]: Same as CICUTA.

Conserve: Flowers or fruits of a single plant beaten into a uniform mass with sugar.

CONSOLIDA: 1) Root of comfrey, *Symphytum officinale*. Emollient used on wounds and abscesses. [15] 2) Same as SOLIDAGO.

CONTRAYERVA: Root of *Dorstenia contrajerva* (and other spp.). Alexipharmic (contrayerva means, literally, "counter herb," i.e., an antidote); astringent tonic and diaphoretic. [2,23,29]

CONTRAYERVAE COMPOSITUS, PULVIS: "Compound powder of contrayerva," a mixture of CONTRAYERVA and PULVIS CHELARUM CANCRI COMPOSITUS. Alexipharmic and diaphoretic. [15]

CONTRAYERVA GERMANORUM: "German antidote." Same as VINCETOXICUM.

CONVALLARIA: Roots of Solomon's seal, *Polygonatum biflorum* and related spp. Used in an anti-inflammatory poultice; other parts of the plant said to be poisonous. [15] Sometimes confused with CONVALLIUM.

CONVALLIUM [LILLIORUM]: Lily of the valley, *Convallaria majalis*. Cephalic and nervine; the roots are said to be errhine. [15] It is now known to contain potentially toxic cardiac glycosides, including convallotoxin, and irritant saponins.

CONVOLVULUS JALAPA: Same as JALAP.

CONVOLVULUS PANDURATUS: Same as MECHOACANNA.

CONVOLVULUS SCAMMONIA: Same as SCAMMONIUM.

CONVOLVULUS SOLDANELLA: See BRASSICA MARINA.

COOK'S PILLS: Compounded of RHEI, ALOE, and CALOMEL, according to an 1830 formula for this proprietary cathartic with cholagogue and emmenagogue properties.

COPAIFERA [OFFICINALIS]: Same as COPAIVA.

COPAIVA (or COPAIBA), [BALSAMUM]: Juice of *Copaifera balsamum*, *C. guyanensis*, or *C. multiyuga*. Brought to Europe from South America by the Portuguese in the 17th century. Tonic to the nervous system; cathartic, diuretic, and antitussive; antivenereal. Side effects include nausea, vomiting, and hematuria. [15,23,29,30]

COPAL: Resin said to come from *Rhus copallinum*, a South American tree, but see RHUS COPALLINUM. Properties unknown. [15]

COPERAS, BLUE: Same as VITRIOL, BLUE.

COPERAS, GREEN: Same as FERRUM VITRIOLATUM.

COPERAS, WHITE: Same as ZINCUM VITRIOLATUM.

COPPER: See CUPRUM.

COPPER PILL: Same as PILULE AMMONIARETI CUPRI.

COPTIS: Same as NIGELLA.

CORALLINA: A form of coral said to be anthelminthic, but probably only absorbent. [15]

CORALLIUM RUBRUM: 1) In the 18th century, red coral, secreted by organisms of genus *Corallium*. Absorbent, corroborant, antidyspeptic, antiepileptic, and astringent, all effects attributable to its calcium carbonate content. [15,23] 2) A preparation of HYDRARGYRUS NITRATUS RUBER invented by Paracelsus in the 16th century (he called it Arcanum Corallinum).

Cordial: A mildly stimulating drug that raises the spirits.

CORDIAL JULEP: Usually a clear, sweet, nonfatty liquid, without sediment, and often containing CAMPHOR among other ingredients. Narcotic. [2]

CORDIA MYXA: See SEBESTENA.

CORIANDRUM [SATIVUM]: Seeds of coriander, *Coriandrum sativum*. Aromatic and carminative. [15,29]

CORNACHINI, PULVIS: Same as POWDER OF THE EARL OF WARWICK; Cornachinus, a professor of medicine at Pisa, was also credited with its invention.

CORNU CERVI[S], SAL: Same as HARTSHORN.

CORNU CERVI[S], SPIRITUS: Sometimes identified as spirits of HARTSHORN, but really same as SPIRITUS AMMONIAE AROMATICUS. Smelling-salts. [15]

CORNUS FLORIDA: Fruit and bark of dogwood, or boxwood, *Cornus florida*. Tonic, astringent, and febrifuge; a possible substitute for CINCHONA. [23,29]

CORNUS SERICEA: Fruit and bark of swamp dogwood, *Cornus sericea*. Properties like those of CORNUS FLORIDA. [23,29]

CORRAL: Same as CORALLINA or CORALLIUM RUBRUM (def. no. 1).

Corroborant: A tonic.

CORROSIVE SUBLIMATE: Same as HYDRARGYRUS MURIATUS CORROSIVUS.

Cortex: A bark or rind (e.g., CORTEX AURANTII is orange peel); but if used with no qualifying adjective, synonymous with CINCHONA.

CORTEX PERUVIANA: Same as CINCHONA.

COSIMO, POWDER OF FATHER: An escharotic based on CINNABAR.

COSMETIC UNGUENT: Made from ARUM MACULATUM. [2]

COSTUMARY: See BALSAMITA.

COSTUS: Perhaps juice of *Costus spicatus* (diuretic) or *Saussurea lappa* (expectorant).

COTULA FOETIDA: Leaves of mayweed, or wild chamomile, *Anthemis cotula*. Said to have same effects as CHAMAEMELUM, but rarely used by late 18th century because of its foul odor. In small doses, tonic and diaphoretic; emetic in large doses; also, antispasmodic, emmenagogue, and a topical vesicant. [15,29,30]

COWHAGE: See DOLICHOS.

COW-PARSNIP: See HERACLEUM SPHONDYLIUM.

CRAB CLAWS, or CRAB'S EYES: See CANCER, CHELAE, and CANCRORUM LAPILLI.

CRANBERRY: See UVA URSI.

CRANESBILL: Same as GERANIUM MACULATUM.

CRATO'S AMBER: A mixture of SUCCINUM, Socotrine ALOES, AGARICUS, ARISTOLOCHIA, and honey made into a pill. Cathartic and antispasmodic.

CREAM OF TARTAR (or CREMOR TARTAR): Powdered sodium potassium tartrate, originally extracted from the dregs (called "tartar") of wine casks. A mild, cooling, and brisk hydragogue cathartic; also, diuretic and deobstruent, especially in fevers. Often combined with other cathartics, e.g., SENNA, JALAP, or ANTIMONIUM TARTARISATUM, to enhance their activity. Sometimes used as a collyrium. [1,2,15,23,29,30]

CREASOTUM: Creosote, volatile oil first obtained by the destructive distillation of wood by German natural philosopher Baron Karl von Reichenbach in 1827. Irritant, narcotic, styptic, antiseptic, and escharotic. Side effects include giddiness, reduced vision, bradycardia, convulsions, and coma. [29]

CRETA: Chalk, calcium carbonate. Antacid, especially for diarrhea. [1,15]

CRETACEUS (or CRETAE COMPOSITUS), PULVIS: "Compound powder of chalk," a mixture of CRETA, CINNAMOMUM, GUM ARABIC, PIPER LONGUM, and NUTMEG or TORMENTILLA. For gastric acidity and accompanying diarrhea. [15]

CRETAE COMPOSITUS CUM OPIO, PULVIS: "Compound powder of chalk and opium," made of CRETA and OPIUM; the latter increases the antidiarrheal effect of the absorbent chalk. [15]

CROCOMAGMA: "Saffron ointment." Same as CONFECTIO DEMOCRATIS.

Crocus: Any yellow or red metallic oxides (i.e., with the color of CROCUS).

CROCUS [SATIVUS]: Stigmas of saffron, *Crocus sativa*. Aromatic, cordial, narcotic, anti-hysteric, and emmenagogue, but of doubtful therapeutic value; also used for yellow coloring. [15,23,29,30]

CROCUS ANTIMONII: See ANTIMONII, CROCUS.

CROCUS MARTIS APERITIVUS: Literally, "iron–rust opener," a heated mixture of FERRI LIMATURA PURIFICATA and SULPHUR (the product is FERRI RUBIGO). Deobstruent and emmenagogue.

CROCUS METALLORUM: Same as ANTIMONII, CROCUS.

CROLL'S STYPTIC PLASTER: Invented by Paracelsian chemist Oswald Croll of Anhalt by 1608. Its 31 ingredients included MINIUM, CALAMINE, WHITE LEAD, BDELLIUM, MUMMY, ANTIMONIUM, HEMATITE, ZINCUM VITRIOLATUM, and MOTHER-OF-PEARL.

CROTON ELEUTHERIA: Same as CASCARILLA.

CROTON OIL: See OLEUM TIGLII.

CROWFOOT: Same as RANUNCULUS.

CRYSTALLI TARTARI: Same as CREAM OF TARTAR.

CRYSTALLUS MINERALIS: Same as SAL PRUNELLAE.

CUBEBA: Cubebs, fruit of the vine *Piper cubeba*. An aromatic stimulant; pectoral; sometimes said to be diuretic. [15,29,30]

CUCKOOPINT: See ARUM MACULATUM.

CUCUMBER: See CUCUMIS AGRESTIS.

CUCUMIS AGRESTIS: Juice from the fruit of wild, or squirting, cucumber, *Ecballium* (or *Momordica*) *elaterium*. Dangerously strong hydragogue cathartic with emetic and diuretic properties. [15,29] Sometimes still used as a cathartic; it irritates the small intestine so as to inhibit the reabsorption of water from the lumen.

CUCUMIS COLOCYNTHIS: Same as COLOCYNTHIS.

CUCURBITA CUM FERRO: "Gourd with iron [blade]," i.e., wet cupping; see BLEEDING.

CUMINUM: Aromatic seeds of *Cuminum cyminum*. Used in plasters and cataplasms. [15]

CUNILA: American dittany, *Cunila origanoides*. Febrifuge.

CUPPA EMETICA: Emetic cup, made of ANTIMONIUM VITRIFICATUM; when wine stands in it for a day or two, it takes on the emetic property of the antimony.

CUPRI VITRIOLATI COMPOSITA, AQUA: Solution of BLUE VITRIOL and ALUM. Styptic, for external use. [15,23]

CUPRUM: Copper. The metal was not used in medicine, but many of its salts were. Because most of them are violently emetic and produce serious central nervous system stimulation, they were seldom used in oral preparations. The dangers of drinking acid liquids that had been stored in copper vessels were well understood. See, e.g., CUPRUM AMMONIACUM and VITRIOL, BLUE. [15,23; also see ref. 8, pp. 65–68]

CUPRUM AMMONIACUM: "Ammoniated copper," a pill made of AMMONIA PRAEPARATA and BLUE VITRIOL. Used to inhibit "moving fibers" in epilepsy, but seldom effective. [1,15,23]

CURARE: See PAREIRA BRAVA.

CURCUMA [LONGA]: Root of turmeric, *Curcuma longa*. Tonic, aperient, emmenagogue, aromatic, and, because it turns the urine reddish-yellow, anti-icteric. [2,15,23,29,30] Also used in curry powders.

CURCUMA ZEDOARIA: See ZEDOARIA.

CURRANTS: See RIBES NIGRA, RIBES RUBRUM, and UVAE PASSAE.

CURSUTA: Root of cursuta, once called *Gentina purpurea*, but probably same as GENTIAN.

CYCLAMEN: See ARTHANITA.

CYDONIA MALUS: Fruit and seeds of quince, *Cydonia oblonga*. Used as an antiemetic and mild cathartic because it is acid and mucilaginous; the wood is astringent. [15]

CYMINUM: Same as CUMINUM.

Cynanchica: Sore throat remedies.

CYNOGLOSSUS: Root of hound's tongue, *Cynoglossum officinale*. Narcotic, antispasmodic, sedative, astringent, and expectorant. [15]

CYNOSBATUS: Fruit (hips) of dog rose, *Rosa caninus*. Used as a binding agent for various drugs, in, e.g., conserves; also, a cooling restringent. [15,23]

CYPERUS: Root of a marsh grass, *Cyperus longus*. Stomachic and carminative. [15]

Cyphi: Aromatic troches.

CYPRESS POWDER: A cosmetic unguent made with ARUM MACULATUM.

CYTISUS: See GENISTA and SCOPARIUS.

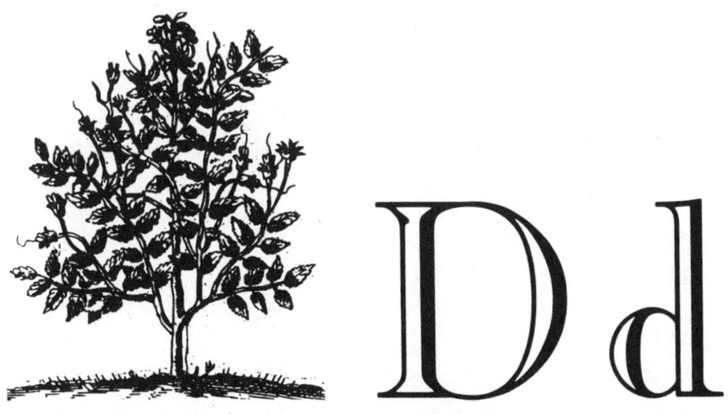

Dd

Dictamnus albus

DACTYLUS: Date, fruit of *Phoenix dactylifera*. Emollient, incrassating, and slightly astringent; used chiefly in pectoral decoctions. [15]

DAFFY'S ELIXIR: Invented by Rev. Thomas Daffy about 1650, and marketed, beginning about 1673, by Anthony Daffy in London as "Elixir Salutis" (i.e., "Elixir of Health") for gout, stone, colic, "ptissick," scurvy, dropsy, rickets, and "languishing and melancholly."The original ingredients included SENNA, CARUM, CARDAMOMUM MINUS, raisins, and alcohol. Never patented, it was a cathartic and diuretic panacea sold by a number of competing firms (and Daffy relatives), and many healers made up their own versions, adding other ingredients, e.g., GLYCERRHIZA. Later admitted to pharmacopoeias as TINCTURA SENNAE COMPOSITA. [14,15]

DALBY'S CARMINATIVE: Invented about 1781 by a London apothecary, J. Dalby, but not patented. An antidiarrheal, it was promoted for "Disorders of the Bowels." An 1824 reconstruction of the unknown original formula included OPIUM and MAGNESIA. [14]

DAMOCRATIS, CONFECTIO: Same as DEMOCRATIS, CONFECTIO.

DANDELION: See TARAXACUM.

DAPHNE MEZEREUM: Same as MEZEREUM.

DATE: See DACTYLUS.

DATURA STRAMONIUM: Same as STRAMONIUM.

DAUCUS CAROTA: Same as DAUCUS SYLVESTRIS.

DAUCUS CRETICUS: Seeds of candy carrot, *Athamanta cretensis*. Carminative and diuretic. [15]

DAUCUS SYLVESTRIS: Seeds of Queen-Anne's lace, or common wild carrot, *Daucus carota*. Used chiefly in cataplasms; also, carminative, diuretic, antiscorbutic, and anthelminthic. [15,23,29,30]

DEADLY NIGHTSHADE: See BELLADONNA.

DE CITRO, TABELLAE: A cathartic electuary made with CITRUS rind.

Decoction or Decoctum: An extract obtained by boiling the raw plant ingredient(s) in water.

DELLA LENA'S POWDER OF MARS: A proprietary remedy made with FERRUM TARTARISATUM, patented in 1799.

DELPHINIUM: Root of larkspur, *Delphinium* spp. Diuretic, emmenagogue, and vermifuge; vulnerary, when applied topically. [29] Also see STAPHISAGRIA.

DE MEL: See MEL.

DEMOCRATIS, CONFECTIO: Confection of Democrates; sometimes based on CROCUS SATIVUS, but sometimes same as MITHRIDATE. Attributed to the 5th-century B.C. Greek scholar Democritus of Abdera.

DE MORBO: Same as NEAPOLITAN UNGUENT.

Demulcent: An agent that prevents the action of acrid and stimulant materials by lubricating the surface exposed to them with a mild viscid matter. Used for, e.g., catarrh, diarrhea, dysentery, renal calculi, and gonorrhea (i.e., spermatorrhea), and in some poultices.

DENS LEONIS: See TARAXACUM.

Dentilavium: A medicated mouthwash.

Deobstruent: A drug that removes obstructions, usually to facilitate the free flow of urine, sweat, feces, phlegm, bile, and blood.

DESICCATIVUM RUBRUM, UNGUENT: "Red desiccating ointment," made with WHITE LEAD, LINIMENT CERATE, ARMENIAN BOLE, and CAMPHOR. [2]

DE SUCCO ROSARUM, TABELLAE: "Tablets of rose juice," a cathartic and cholagogue electuary made with AQUA ROSARUM.

Detergent: A medicine that cleanses or purges.

Detersive: Detergent.

Dia—: Prefix denoting something prescribed by a physician; in most of the immediately following entries (through DIAZINGIBER), the prefix denotes a compound medicine.

DIABORACIS: An antihysteric powder made with BORAX.

DIABOTANUM: A plaster made with many different plants.

DIABRYONIAS, ELECTUARIUM: A cephalic and mildly cathartic remedy made with BRYONIA.

DIABRYONIAS, UNGUENTUM: An unguent, with cathartic properties, made with BRYONIA, CUCUMIS, SCILLA, ARUM MACULATUM, EBULUS, IRIS FLORENTINA, and an unspecified fern; also see UNGUENTUM AGRIPPAE.

DIABUGLOSSI: A cardiac powder made with BUGLOSSUM.

DIACALAMINTHES: A complex stomachic, carminative, and antihysteric powder based on CALAMINE.

DIACARION: Same as DIANUCUM.

DIACARTHAMI: A cathartic and expectorant electuary made with CARTHAMUS.

DIACASSIA: Same as ELECTUARIUM CASSIAE.

DIACASTOREUM: A cephalic and antihysteric electuary made with CASTOREUM.

DIACATHOLICON: A complex cathartic panacea based on CASSIA and SENNA.

DIACHALCITEOS: Same as EMPLASTRUM DIAPALMA.

DIACHYLON, EMPLASTRUM: Common plaster made with WHITE LEAD and OL OLIVA. Used to protect broken skin. [2]

DIACINNABARIS: An antiepileptic powder made with CINNABAR.

DIACINNAMOMI: A cordial and stomachic powder made with CINNAMOMUM or CANELLA.

DIACNICUM: Syrup of CARTHAMUS.

DIACODIUM: A weak aqueous solution of 6% OPIUM of which 0.7 oz. produced the same effect as 1 gr. SOLID PANACEA. [2,3] In U.S., made with heads of PAPAVER ALBUM.

DIACORUM: A complex cephalic electuary made with CALAMUS AROMATICUS.

DIACRETAE: An astringent powder made with CRETA.

DIACROCUM: A tonic, diaphoretic, and antihysteric powder made with CROCUS.

DIACRYDIUM: A preparation made with SCAMMONIUM.

DIACRYSTALLI: A lactagogue powder of unknown composition.

DIACYMINI: A cephalic, antihysteric, and stomachic powder made with CUMINUM.

DIADAMASCENUM CHOLAGOGUM: Same as DIAPRUNUM SOLITIVUM.

DIADICTAMNUM CERATUM: A vulnerary liniment made with DICTAMNUS ALBUS.

DIAFARFARAE: Pectoral pills made with TUSSILAGO.

DIAGALANGAE: A stomachic and antihysteric powder made with GALANGA MINOR.

DIAGREDIUM: Same as SCAMMONIUM. [Also see ref. 10, p. 57]

DIAHYSSOPI: A stomachic and antiasthmatic powder made with HYSSOPUS.

DIAIREOS: A pectoral and antiasthmatic powder made with IRIS FLORENTINA.

DIAJALAPAE: A cathartic and hydragogue powder made with JALAP.

DIALACCAE: An antihysteric tonic made with LACCA.

DIALAURI: A carminative and antihysteric powder made with LAURUS.

DIALTHEA, UNGUENT: An ointment made with ALTHEA.

DIALUNAE: An antiepileptic powder made with ARGENTUM.

DIAMANNA[E]: A mildly cathartic electuary made with MANNA.

DIAMARGARITUM: A cordial tonic powder made with MARGARITA.

DIAMARGARITUM SIMPLEX: DIAMARGARITUM rolled in sugar.

DIAMERA: A cordial, cephalic, and stomachic powder made with SPERMACETI.

DIAMERCURII: An anthelminthic powder made with HYDRARGYRUS.

DIAMORUM COMPOSITUM: Rob of MORUS mixed with MEL, SAPA, VERDEGRIS, MYRRH, and CROCUS.

DIAMORUM SIMPLEX: Syrup of MORUS.

DIAMORUSIA: A stomachic and antihysteric electuary made with DIAMORUM COMPOSITUM.

DIAMOSCHI DULCIS: A cordial tonic powder made with MOSCHUS.

DIAMPHOLYX, UNGUENTUM: Made with ZINCUM USTUM, WHITE LEAD, juice of BELLADONNA, and OLIBANUM.

DIAMUMIAE: A tonic powder made with pulverized MUMMY.

DIANISI: A digestive, carminative, and antihysteric powder made with ANISUM.

DIANITRI: A diuretic powder made with SAL NITER.

DIANTHOS: A cephalic powder made with ROSMARINUS.

DIANTHUS: See CARYOPHYLLUM RUBRUM.

DIANUCUM: A rob made with juice of green walnuts (see JUGLANS CINEREA) and honey.

DIAOLIBANI: An antiepileptic powder made with OLIBANUM.

DIAPALMA, EMPLASTRUM: A desiccating plaster made of PALMA, WHITE LEAD, OL OLIVA, and water. [2]

DIAPEPEREOS, CERATUM: A wound ointment made with PIPER NIGRUM.

DIAPHAENICUM: A cathartic, antihysteric, and expectorant electuary made with DACTYLUS.

Diaphoretic: A drug that increases natural exhalation through the skin, by directly or indirectly enhancing the tone of the cutaneous blood vessels. Used, e.g., for fever, dropsy, asthma, dyspepsia, chronic diarrhea, and rheumatism.

DIAPHORETIC ANTIMONY: Same as CROCUS ANTIMONII.

DIAPHORETIC MIXTURE: A SALINE JULAP (q.v.).

DIAPHORETIC SALT: Same as AMMONIA PRAEPARATA.

DIAPHORETICUM JOVIALE: Diaphoretic powder made from STANNUM and ANTIMONIUM CALCINATUM.

DIAPHORETICUM MINERALE: Same as ANTIMONIUM TARTARISATUM.

DIAPHORETICUM SOLARE: A preparation made with AURUM and an ANTIMONY salt. Also a stomachic.

DIAPLANTAGINIS: An astringent powder made with PLANTAGO.

DIAPOMPHOLIGOS, UNGUENTUM: Made of POMPHOLYX, BELLADONNA berry juice, WHITE LEAD, and RED LEAD. For skin ulcers.

DIAPRASSII: A complex cephalic powder based on MARRUBIUM.

DIAPRUNUM SIMPLEX: A cathartic electuary based on PRUNUS.

DIAPRUNUM SOLITIVUM: A cathartic electuary based on PRUNUS and SCAMMONIUM.

DIAPYRITES: A vulnerary liniment made with pyrites ("fool's gold," iron sulfide).

DIARHODON ABBATIS: A cordial stomachic powder based on ROSA; said to have been invented by the abbot of a medieval monastery.

DIARHODON, PILULE: A cathartic and stomachic pill based on ROSA.

DIARHODON, TROCHISI: Cordial, stomachic, and astringent troches based on dried ROSA.

DIASARUM: A mild cathartic and emetic electuary made with ASARUM.

DIASATURNI: An antiasthmatic and antiphthisic powder made with salts of PLUMBUM and ANTIMONIUM.

DIASCORDIUM: A preparation invented by Girolamo Fracastoro in the early 16th century as a plague remedy that included SCORDIUM (hence the name). By 1700 it included 0.13% OPIUM, containing 1.0-4.1 mg. morphine per recommended dose, depending on body weight, and about 16 other ingredients. [3,13]

DIASEBESTEN: A gentle cathartic electuary made with SEBESTENA.

DIASENNA: A cathartic powder based on SENNA.

DIASENNAE: A cathartic and melanagogue electuary based on SENNA.

DIASPERMATUM: A mixture made with many different kinds of seeds.

DIASUCCINI: An astringent and narcotic powder based on OL SUCCINI.

DIASULPHURIS: 1) An antiasthmatic powder based on

SULPHUR. 2) An antihysteric and somnifacient based on SULPHUR (and, perhaps, OPIUM).

DIASULPHURIS, CERATUM (or EMPLASTRUM): A vulnerary based on SULPHUR.

DIASULPHURIS, TABELLA: Antiasthmatic tablet based on SULPHUR.

DIATAMARON: A stomachic powder based on DACTYLUS.

DIATARTARI [OF CASTELLI]: A cathartic and hydragogue powder based on CREAM OF TARTAR; it also included SENNA, MANNA, ZINGIBER, CINNAMOMUM, and red sugar. Invented by Pietro Castelli of Messina in the 17th century.

DIATESSARON: A complex electuary made with GENTIAN, LAURUS, JUNIPERUS, ARISTOLOCHIA, and honey.

DIATRAGACANTI [FRIGIDI]: An agglutinating and pectoral powder made with GUM TRAGACANTH, GUM ARABIC, ALTHAEA, GLYCERRHIZA, etc.

DIATRIUM PIPERUM: A digestive powder based on PIPER NIGRUM.

DIATRIUM SANTALORUM: A cordial tonic powder based on SANTALUM species.

DIATURBITH: A cathartic, expectorant, and hydragogue powder (or electuary) based on TURPETHUM.

DIATURBITH MINERALE: An emetic electuary based on HYDRARGYRUS VITRIOLATUS.

DIAZINGIBER: A stomachic, carminative, and digestive powder based on ZINGIBER.

DIAZINGIBER LAXATIVUM: A cathartic and expectorant electuary containing ZINGIBER.

DICTAMNUS ALBUS: Leaves of dittany of Crete, *Origanum dictamnus*. Aromatic oil of no special medical utility. [15]

DIET: Often used as specific therapy. For example, at the Royal Infirmary of Edinburgh, Dr. Andrew Duncan, Sr., upgraded the standard "low" (i.e., depletive or antiphlogistic) diet given to all newly admitted patients to "milk" diets for 17% of his 65 teaching patients in 1795, and to "full" diets for another 14%, almost all within a week of their admissions. Another 31% were allowed "meat" or "a bit of meat," and a few more beef tea, after longer intervals, generally during convalescence. Duncan prescribed more nutritious (i.e.,

DIET ITEM	WEEKLY TOTALS FOR PATIENTS ON:		
	LOW DIET	MILK DIET	FULL DIET
Breakfast			
Water-Gruel and/or Milk Pottage (1¼ oz oatmeal in 1 pt water or milk, with raisins added)	7 pt	7 pt	7 pt
Dinner			
Boiled Beef or Mutton, with Greens	0.25 lb	—	2 lb
Roast Veal	0.25 lb	—	—
Rice Milk (rice added to milk to desired consistency)	2 pt	3 pt	1 pt
Boiled Pudding (1 lb flour, ¼ lb suet or meat or eels, fruits, etc., mixed with 13 oz water, tied in bag and boiled 1-2 hr)	—	—	0.5 lb
Bread Pudding (½ lb bread crumbs soaked overnight in 1 pt milk, add 2-3 eggs and salt, tie in bag and boil 1-1½ hr; eat with salt, sugar)	2 lb*	1 lb	—
Broth (leg of lamb or other meat boiled 1½ hr, thickening added, perhaps butter)	2 pt	—	—
Plum Broth (6 oz meat or bone, ½ pt peas, and ½ oz oats, boiled in water)	1 pt	—	1 pt
Plumb Pottage (½ lb bread crumbs soaked in milk, 4 eggs, 1 teacup molasses, lemon brandy or water, few raisins or 4 plums, cinnamon; boil or bake 2 hrs)	—	4 pt	—

Supper			
Broth (see above)	4 pt	—	4 pt
Water-Gruel (see above)	1 pt	7 pt**	1 pt
Cheese or Butter	0.25 lb	—	0.25 lb
DAILY			
Bread, 14-oz loaf	6.125 lb	6.125 lb	6.125 lb
Milk	—	7 pt	—
Beer, Small (i.e., weak or inferior)	7 pt***	—	28 pt****
Water	—	14 pt	—
FOOD TOTALS***** (lb-pts/week)	25.9	35.1	22.9
DAILY AVERAGE***** (lb-pts/week)	3.7	5.0	3.3

* Interpolated estimate; the actual weight may have been less.

** Or, milk pottage

*** 14 pints were allowed from Lady Day, 25 March, through Michaelmas, 21 September.

**** 21 pints were allowed from Lady Day through Michaelmas.

***** Excluding beer and water.

N.B.: Patients receiving mercurial drugs and a low diet were given, in addition, 7 qt. of milk and 3.5 lb. of boiled mutton each week, to counteract the dysgeusic effects of mercury.

SOURCE: *A Table of Diet*, an anonymous late eighteenth-century booklet of six pages of practical instructions bound with Dr. John Jeffries's copy of Joanne Berkenhout, *Pharmacopoeia Medici*, 3rd ed. (London: R. Baldwin, 1782), in the Boston Medical Library, call no. 22.K.7.

stimulant) diets for patients suffering from severe fevers accompanied by specific weaknesses (e.g., paralysed limbs), skin diseases, blood loss (e.g., hemoptysis), and conditions requiring strengthening of the gastrointestinal tract (e.g., dyspepsia). He also prescribed stronger diets for patients convalescing from debilitating fevers. [1] Three late 18th-century hospital diets, and typical contemporary recipes for individual items in them, are given in the accompanying table. [Also see: J. C. Drummond and Anne Wilbraham, *The Englishman's Food*, rev. ed. (London: Jonathan Cape, 1957)]

DIET DRINK: See DECOCTUM SARSAPARILLAE COMPOSITUM.

Digestive: 1) In English usage, a drug that improves digestion and, therefore, nutrition; often also cathartic. 2) In Continental usage, a liquid unguent that encourages wounds to suppurate.

DIGESTIVUM SYLVII, SAL: "Digestive salt of Sylvius;" same as CAPUT MORTUUM; used in sense of def. no. 2 for Digestive. Attributed to 17th–century physician Franz de le Boë, also called Franciscus Sylvius, of Leiden.

DIGESTIVUM, UNGUENTUM: Digestive (def. no. 2) ointment made with OL TEREBINTHA VENETA and egg yolks. [15]

DIGITALIS [PURPUREA]: Powdered leaves of purple foxglove, *Digitalis purpurea*. Introduced to modern medicine by Dr. William Withering of Birmingham, England, 1775-1785. Acts on kidneys as a stimulant diuretic that removes abnormal tissue fluids in dropsy, but also possibly a narcotic that calms the cardiovascular system (thus rendering it suitable for the treatment of consumption). Side effects include vomiting, slow pulse, vertigo, and altered vision. [1,4,23,29,30; for its introduction to modern medical practice, as the result of what was probably the only large controlled clinical trial carried out before 1850 (or even, perhaps, 1940), see: William Withering, *An Account of the Foxglove* (Birmingham: M. Swinney, 1785), and ref. 4, pp. 165-223]. In 1844, Homolle found the active principle, digitaline, later renamed digitoxin, in foxglove leaves, from which it was isolated by Nativelle in 1869.

DILL: See ANETHUM.

Diluent: An agent that increases the proportion of fluid in the blood, or that decreases blood viscosity; synergistic with diuretics and diaphoretics. Used in acute inflammatory diseases, but in a secondary role.

Dinairus: A digestive, in sense of def. no. 2.

DINNER PILLS: A 19th-century proprietary cathartic made with ALOES, MASTICHE, ROSAE, and syrup of ABSINTHUM.

DIOSMA: Same as BUCHU.

DIOSPOLITICON: An antihysteric and emmenagogue powder named for a town in Egypt.

DIOSPYROS: Bark of persimmon tree, *Diospyros* spp. Bitter astringent; anthelminthic. [29,30]

DIPPEL'S ANIMAL OIL: Same as ANIMAL OIL.

Discutient: A medicine that dissipates, dispels, or dissolves morbid matter.

DITTANY, AMERICAN: See CUNILA.

DITTANY OF CRETE: See DICTAMNUS ALBUS.

Diuretic: A drug that promotes urinary discharge, independently of the volume of fluid ingested, by stimulating the secreting vessels of the kidney, or by promoting absorption of tissue fluids by vessels throughout the body (thus enhancing their delivery to the kidneys for excretion). Used for dropsy, urinary calculi, gonorrhea (i.e., spermatorrhea), and excessive sweating. DIGITALIS, introduced in 1785, was the first dependable apparent diuretic (at least for dropsy patients).

DIURETIC SALT: Usually, same as ACETIS POTASSAE. Diuretic and cathartic. [2]

DIVINUM EMPLASTRUM: A tonic vulnerary plaster named for its wonderful effects.

DIXON'S [ANTIBILIOUS] PILLS: A 19th-century proprietary cathartic made with ALOES, SCAMMONIUM, RHEI, and ANTIMONIUM TARTARISATUM.

DOCK, CURLY-LEAVED: Same as RUMEX CRISPUS.

DOCK, NARROW-LEAVED: Same as RUMEX ACUTUS.

DOCK, WATER: See HYDROLAPATHUM.

DOGBANE, SPREADING: See APOCYNUM ANDROSAEMIFOLIUM.

DOG ROSE: See CYNOSBATUS.

DOG'S BANE: See APOCYNUM CANNABINUM.

DOGWOOD: See CORNUS FLORIDA and CORNUS SERICEA.

DOLICHOS [PRURIENS]: The stiff down on the pods of

cowhage, *Mucuna pruriens.* A tropical American plant first described in 1640 and promoted as a medicine in England from 1769. Anthelminthic. [15,23,29]

DORONIUM GERMANICUM: "German gift." Same as ARNICA MONTANA.

DORSTENIA CONTRAYERVA: Same as CONTRAYERVA.

Dose and Dosage: Some drugs were readily recognized to be more potent than others of the same class and, therefore, to require a smaller dose in order to produce an equivalent effect. Additional factors taken into account included: body weight and habitus [see, for an example, ref. 3]; sex ("Women, in general, require smaller doses of any medicine than men, a difference probably owing to their greater sensibility from their habits of life" [ref. 23, p. 576]); the symptoms to be treated; habituation to the drug (e.g., OPIUM); and, especially, age. However, idiosyncratic reactions to drugs (i.e., those not predictable from any factor listed above), were also recognized [ref. 23, pp. 575-577]. The following table gives proportional doses for people of increasing age, using the conventional dose for a typical "middle aged person" as the standard (i.e., = 1):

1 year	= 1/12	4–7 years	= 1/3
2 years	= 1/8	7–14 years	= 1/2
3 years	= 1/6	14–21 years	= 2/3
4 years	= 1/4		

DOVER'S POWDER: Originally a mixture of one part each of OPIUM, IPECAC, and GLYCERRHIZA, and four parts each of SAL NITER and KALI SULPHURATUM, administered in white wine, that was introduced in 1732 by Dr. Thomas Dover of Bristol and London as a diaphoretic for treating rheumatic complaints and dropsy. It was later simplified to include only equal parts of OPIUM and IPECAC (although KALI SULPHURATUM was sometimes added because its grittiness helped to further pulverize the resinous opium during the mixing process), and used chiefly as a diaphoretic. [1,2,23; also see Kenneth Dewhurst, *Thomas Dover's Life and Legacy* (New York: Academy of Medicine, 1974)].

Drachm (or Dram): See Measurement.

DRACONTIUM FOETIDUM: Same as ARUM AMERICANUM.

DRAGON ROOT: See ARUM MACULATUM.

DRAGON'S BLOOD: See SANGUIS DRACONIS.

DRASTRICUM, EXTRACTUM: An extract of SCAMMONY in juice of AURANTIUM.

Drop[s]: See Measurement.

Dropax: A depilatory plaster.

DROPWORT: See OENANTHE.

DULCAMARA: "Bittersweet," because of the taste of the stalks or berries of European bittersweet, or climbing nightshade, *Solanum dulcamara*. Introduced to medicine in Germany in mid-16th century. Diaphoretic, diuretic, cathartic, discutient, emmenagogue, antimanic, and antaphrodisiac. May produce narcotic effects like those of BELLADONNA, but less potent. [15,23,29] The active antimuscarinic alkaloid, solanine, was isolated by Desfosses in 1820.

DULCIFIED SPIRIT[S] OF NITRE, or SPIRIT[S] OF NITROUS ETHER: SPIRIT OF NITER in alcohol. Refrigerant, tonic, diaphoretic, diuretic, and antispasmodic. [2,23]

DULCIFIED SPIRIT OF SALT: Prepared by heating equal parts of ACIDUM MURIATICUM and VINUM. Diuretic, febrifuge, and alexipharmic.

DULCIFIED SPIRIT OF VITRIOL: Same as AETHER SULPHURICUS CUM ALCOHOLE.

DUOBUS, SAL DE: "Two-part salt;" same as KALI SULPHURATUM.

DUTCH DROPS: Invented by Claas Tilly of Haarlem in 1672. Made with TEREBINTHA; another brand added GUIAC, SPIRIT OF NITER, OL SUCCINI, and OL CARYOPHYLLUS AROMATICUS. [13] The 20th-century version, used for skin ailments, is made with OL JUNIPERUS.

Dysenteric: A drug for dysentery.

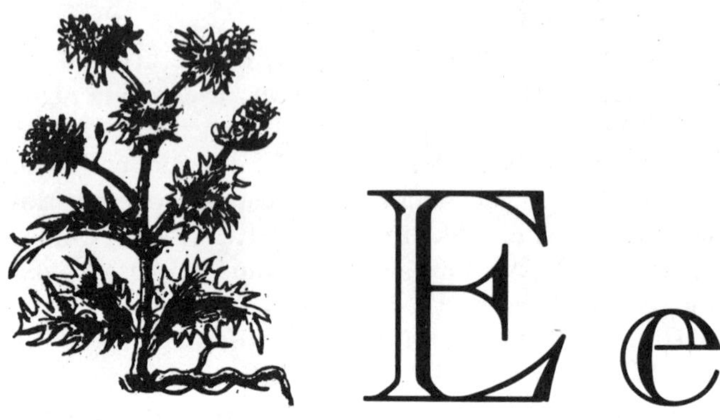

Eryngium

EBULUS: Root, leaves, and berries of dwarf elder, *Sambucus ebulus*. Strong cathartic. [15]

ECBALLIUM: See CUCUMIS AGRESTIS.

Ecbolia: Remedies that expel dead fetuses from the uterus.

Eccoprotica: Laxatives that cause a gentle emesis before they rectify the humors.

Eclegma: Expectorant remedies with the consistency of a thick syrup, to be sucked by the patient from the end of a licorice root (see GLYCERRHIZA).

Ecphractica: Remedies that close and dry the body's pores, e.g., drugs with antidiuretic or antidiaphoretic properties.

Ectylotica: Remedies that dissolve calluses.

Ecusson: A plaster made of THERIAC with added OPIUM.

Edulcorant: A sweetening or softening agent.

EFFERVESCING DRAUGHT: Same as LIQUOR POTASSAE CITRATIS.

EGGS: See OVUM.

EGYPTIACUM, MEL: "Egyptian honey." Same as OXYMEL AERUGINIS.

EGYPTIACUM, UNGUENTUM: "Egyptian ointment."

Made of VERDEGRIS, ACETUM, and honey (but not a true unguent, since it contained no oils or fats). Variations on this formula included additional astringent ingredients (e.g., ALUM). Escharotic. [2]

EGYPTIAN MIMOSA: Same as GUM ARABIC.

ELAPI: Same as HARTSHORN.

ELATERIUM: Same as CUCUMIS AGRESTIS.

ELDER: See EBULUS.

ELDERBERRY: See SAMBUCUS.

ELECAMPANE: See ENULA CAMPANA.

ELECTRICITY: Discharges from static electricity generators were first used therapeutically, for treating paralyzed patients, by Dr. Christian Gottlieb Kratzenstein in 1745. Luigi Galvani's 1786 discovery that living tissues possess electrical properties provided a further stimulus for the clinical application of electricity, as did Alessandro Volta's invention of the pile battery in 1799. In 1813 Dr. James Thacher of Plymouth, Mass., succinctly summarized current clinical thinking about medical electricity: "The medicinal operation of electricity may be refered to its stimulant power. It produces forcible contractions in the irritable fibre; excites therefore to action if duly applied; and when in excess, immediately exhausts irritability. It possesses the important advantage of being easily brought to act locally, and of being confined to the part to which it is applied, while it can also be employed in every degree of force.

"Electricity is applied to the body under the form of a stream or continued discharge of the fluid, under that of sparks, and under that of shock; the first being more gentle, the second more active, and the last much more powerful than either of the others. The stream is applied by connecting a pointed piece of wood, or a metal wire, with the prime conductor of the electrical machine, and holding it by a glass handle, one or two inches from the part, to which it is to be directed. A very moderate stimulant action is thus excited, which is better adapted to some particular cases, than the more powerful spark or shock.

"The spark is drawn by placing the patient on the insulated stool, connected with the prime conductor, and, while the machine is worked, bringing a metal knob within a short distance of the part, from which the spark is to be taken. A sensation somewhat pungent is excited, and slight muscular contractions may be produced; these effects being greater or less, according to the distance at which the knob is held, if the machine be sufficiently powerful.

"The shock is given by discharging the Leyden [jar], making the part of the body, through which it is intended to be transmitted, part of the circuit. The sensation it excites is unpleasant, and the muscular contraction considerable, if the shock be moderately strong.

"The general rule for the medical employment of electricity, is to apply it at first under the milder forms, and gradually to raise it, if necessary, to the more powerful. Mr. Cavallo . . . finds it most efficacious to expose the patient to the electrical aura discharged from an iron or wooden point; or, if shocks be given, they should be very slight, and not exceed thirteen or fourteen at a time . . . The patient may be electrified from three to ten minutes; but, if sparks be drawn, they should not exceed the number of shocks above mentioned." [23, pp. 587-588]

Another method of applying therapeutic electricity was provided by the Voltaic pile, or battery, consisting of alternating plates of silver (or copper) and zinc (or tin) stacked in a strong solution of NITER, SAL AMMONIACUS, or SAL MURIATICUS, and connected by wires to the part of the body to be treated. The shock induced by such apparatus was thought to be analogous to that produced by the electric eel or torpedo, and its strength was proportional to the size of the pile. [23, pp. 592-594; also, for the relation of medical to marine electricity, see Chan H. Wu, "Electric Fish and the Discovery of Animal Electricity," *American Scientist 72* (1984): 598-607]

According to Thacher, the illnesses most amenable to treatment by electricity included: rheumatic disorders, deafness, toothache, non-purulent swellings, ophthalmias, palsies, cutaneous ulcers and eruptions, open sores, lock-jaw, nervous headache, and amenorrhea, although not all of these conditions responded equally well. [23, pp. 588-591] Other physicians recommended electricity most often simply to "relieve torpor" in nerves to specific muscles or organs that had long been paralyzed. For instance, it was applied over the kidneys of diabetics, to induce constriction of their renal arteries and thus reduce their urine output. [1; also see J. C. Carpue, *An Introduction to Electricity and Galvanism* (London: A. Phillips, 1803)]. Carpue noted that "electricity increases the natural evaporation of animals, &c.," and so might find use in dropsy.

Electuary: A medicinal paste or lozenge consisting of powder mixed with honey, to make a thick paste with a consistency suitable for taking up a dose on the tip of a knife. Used chiefly for administering mild drugs, because of the uncertainty of actually ingesting an exactly prescribed dose of hazardous drugs administered in electuaries.

ELEMI: Gum elemi, resin from any of several trees, e.g., *Canarium commune*, *Icaca icicariba*, and *Elaphrium elemiferum*. Stimulant tonic; also used in plasters and ointments. [15,29]

ELETTERIA: See CARDAMOMUM MINUS.

ELEUTHERIA: Same as CASCARILLA.

Elixir: A sweetened aromatic alcoholic drug extract.

ELM: See ULMUS entries.

Embrocation: An ointment to be rubbed into painful body parts; a liniment.

EMERALDS: See LIMONATA SMARAGDINA.

Emetic: A drug that excites vomiting, probably via an effect on the brain and nerves, but not on the stomach; may promote absorption, catharsis, or diaphoresis in lower doses. Used for conditions accompanied by fever, distention of the stomach, hyperacidity, poisoning, intoxication, biliary jaundice, or dropsy, among others.

EMETIC TARTAR: Same as ANTIMONIUM TARTARISATUM.

EMETICUS, PULVIS: "Emetic powder," same as ALGAROTH'S POWDER.

EMETIC WEED: See LOBELIA INFLATA.

EMETIC WINE: Same as VINUM ANTIMONII.

Emmenagogue: A drug that promotes menstrual discharge by stimulating uterine vessels, or by virtue of its antihysteric properties. Used in, e.g., amenorrhea. Also see Antihysteric.

Emmota: Liquid liniments that prevent pustules (e.g., those of smallpox) from leaving permanent scars.

Emollient: A drug that reduces the cohesion between particles of solid matter in the body by lessening the friction between them, especially when the tissues are rigid or distended. By the mid-19th century, emollients were understood to be vehicles for applying warmth and moisture, while excluding air from the diseased tissue beneath. Used, e.g., to treat tumors, inflammations, and dryness of the skin.

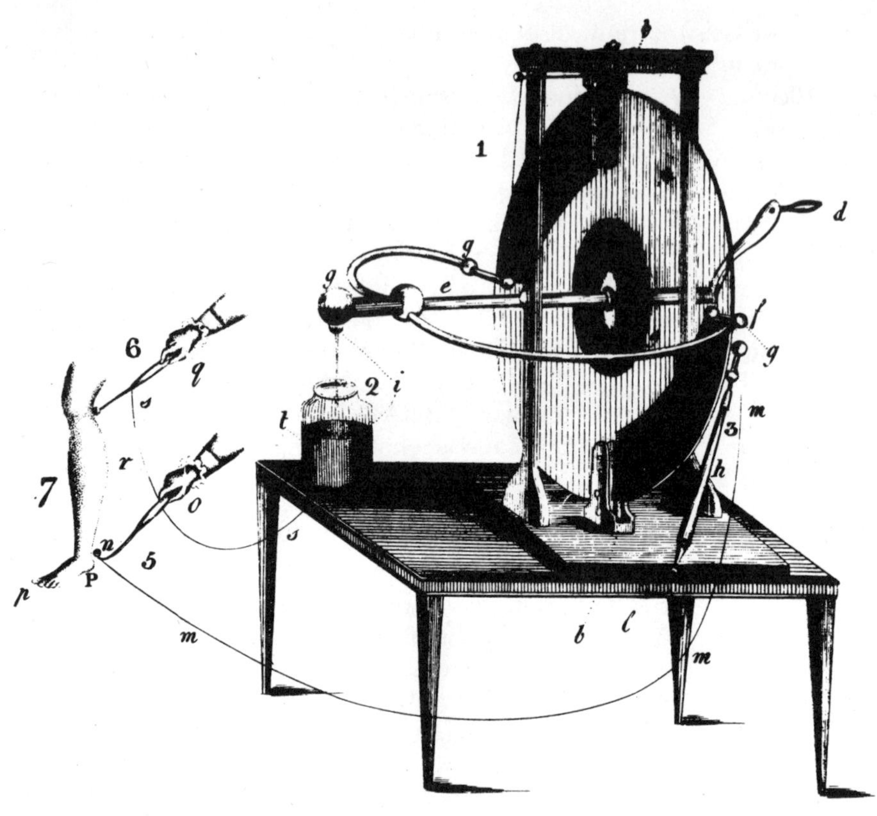

Fig. 1 (above): STATIC ELECTRICITY GENERATOR, being used to stimulate a paralyzed leg. The large glass wheel was turned by the handle (d) so as to be "excited" by the "rubbers," the two large dark areas covering opposite quadrants on the periphery of the wheel; they were made of leather impregnated with a mercury amalgam and lined with the silk which actually generated the electrical charges. The dark circle in the center of the wheel represents brass bushings on either side of the whell, which was insulated from the rest of the machine by a glass cylinder (e). The curved brass "prime conductor" tubing (g,g,g) received the "electric fluid" from the wheel; the balls along the conductor's course prevented spontaneous loss of fluid, which was collected in the Leyden jar (2). The electrometer (3) was adjusted to regulate the strength of the shock administered to the patient.

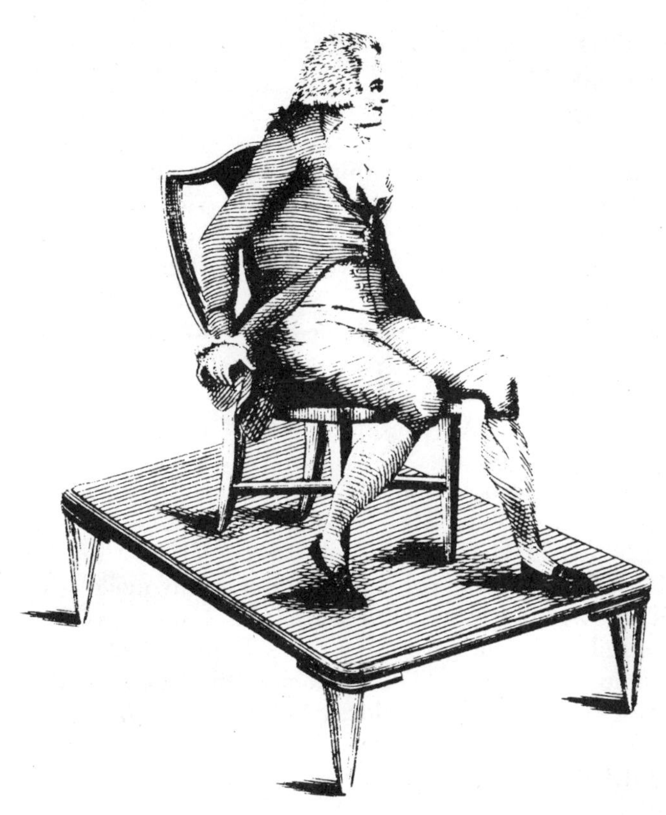

Applying glass-handled "directors" (5,6) so that their brass balls, which were connected with, respectively, the electrometer via wire (m) and the outside coating of the leyden jar (t), completed the circuit that resulted in a shock that passed from the heel to the top of the leg. This was called a Cuthbertson-type apparatus. Other models used a glass cylinder rather than a wheel, and some were more suitable for taking to a patient's bedside because they were portable; some were quite compact, and fitted within a wooden box.

Fig. 2 (above): METHOD OF "DRAWING SPARKS" from the leg of a patient seated on an insulated platform, using a generator such as the one shown in Fig. 1.

SOURCE (Figs. 1 and 2): J. C. Carpue, An Introduction to Electricity and Galvanism (London: A. Phillips, Longman and Rees, and Cadell and Davies, 1803), plate 2.

Empasmata: Astringent powders that correct bad breath and excessive sweating.

Emphrastica: Same as Ecphractica.

EMPLASTRUM: See Plaster.

Emplattomena: Plasters with the properties of Ecphratica.

Emulsion: An aqueous suspension of oily and/or resinous materials.

EMULSIO OLEOSA VOLATILIS: See OLEO MIXTURE.

Enaemon: An agglutinating remedy that stops hemorrhage and heals wounds.

Enchiloma: An elixir.

Enchristum: An unguent or liniment.

Enchyta: Eyedrops.

ENDIVIA: Seeds of endive, *Chicorium endivia*, a cooling aperient. [15] Also see CICHOREUM.

ENEMA, DOMESTIC: Usually, SAL MURIATICUS and OL OLIVA in warm water; another was made with ALTHAEA and CHAMAEMELUM. Used to relieve prolonged constipation. [1; also see Julius Friedenwald and Samuel Morrison, "The History of the Enema with Some Notes on Related Procedures," *Bulletin of the History of Medicine 8* (1940): 68-114, 239-276].

ENGLISH POWDER: A preparation of CINCHONA, FOLIA ROSARUM, and SUCCUS LIMONI introduced in France by Sir Robert Talbor (or Talbot) in 1679. Another reported formula included TINCTURA CINCHONAE, SUCCUS PETROSELINUS, and DECOCTUM ANISI.

ENGLISH SALTS: Same as MAGNESIA VITRIOLATA (i.e., Epsom salts, because they came from England).

Ens: A Paracelsian term for the essential, or active, part of a material.

ENS (or ESSENCE) VENERIS: "Essence of Venus," a mixture of SAL AMMONIAC and VITRIOL.

ENULA CAMPANA: Root of elecampane, *Inula helenium*. Expectorant, diuretic, diaphoretic, cathartic, stomachic, and emmenagogue. [15,23,29] Inulin, a fructose-like sugar isolated from it in 1804, is now used to assess glomerular filtration rate.

ENULATUM, UNGUENTUM: An ointment for itch made with ENULA CAMPANA.

Epicarpia: Cataplasms made with sharp, penetrating ingredients, which reduce the heat of local inflammations.

EPILEPTIC POWDER: Same as PULVIS AD GUTTETAM.

Epiplasma: Cataplasms.

Epispastic: A blistering agent; see CANTHARIS.

Epithema: 1) Alcohol fomentations to be applied over the heart and stomach. 2) Moist, soft poultices containing blistering or astringent materials, e.g., SINAPI or SAL MURIATICUS, for the breast, back, or shoulders.

EPSOM SALT: Same as MAGNESIA VITRIOLATA.

Epulotica: Caustic plasters.

ERGOT: See SECALE CORNUTUM.

ERIGERON CANADENSE: Canada fleabane, mule-tail, or horse-weed, *Erigeron* (or *Conyza*) *canadensis*. Tonic, diuretic, and astringent. [29,30]

ERIGERON HETEROPHYLLUM: Daisy fleabane, *Erigeron annuus*. Diuretic. [29]

ERIGERON PHILADELPHICUM: Common, daisy, or Philadelphia fleabane, *Erigeron philadelphicus*. Diuretic. [29]

Errhine: A drug that increases mucus or serous discharge from the nostrils, or that induces sneezing, because of its bitter qualities when applied locally. Used for, e.g., headache, earache, and ophthalmia. [2]

ERUCA: Seeds of rocket, *Eruca sativa*. Aphrodisiac. [15]

ERYNGIUM: Root of water eryngo, or sea holly, *Eryngium maritimum*. Diaphoretic, expectorant, sialagogue, aperient, diuretic, aphrodisiac, and, occasionally, emetic. [15,29,30]

ERYNGO: Common eryngo, *Eryngium campestre*. Aperient, diuretic, aphrodisiac.

ERYSIMUM: See ALLIARIA.

ERYTHRONIUM: Root and whole plant of trout-lily, or adder's-tongue, *Erythronium americanum*. Emetic of doubtful therapeutic value. [29]

Escharotic: A chemical that dissolves or destroys animal matter. Used for skin ulcers and excrescences.

ESSENCE OF PEPPERMINT: Patented by London apothecary John Juniper in 1762 and marketed as a carminative, its basic ingredient was MENTHA PIPERITA. [Olive R. Jones, "Essence of Peppermint, a History of the Medicine and Its Bottle," *Historical Archaeology 15* (1981): 1-57].

ESSENTIAL SALT OF LEMON: A misnomer for potassium oxalate extracted from ACETOSA.

ETHER: See AETHER VITRIOLICUS.

ETHIOPS: See AETHIOPS entries.

EUGENIA CARYOPHYLLATA: Same as CARYOPHYLLUS AROMATICUS.

EUPATORIUM: Hemp agrimony, *Eupatorium cannabinum*. Tonic, aperient, antiscorbutic, cathartic, and narcotic. [15]

EUPATORIUM PERFOLIATUM: Leaves and flowers of thoroughwort, or purple boneset, *Eupatorium perfoliatum*. Tonic, diaphoretic, emetic, cathartic, and febrifuge. [23,29,30]

EUPATORIUM PILOSUM: Leaves of hairy thoroughwort, or wild horehound, *Eupatorium pilosum*. Tonic, diaphoretic, and mildly cathartic. [23]

EUPHORBIA COROLLATA: Root of flowering spurge, *Euphorbia corollata*. Diaphoretic and expectorant in small doses, powerfully cathartic and emetic in large doses; vesicant when applied to the skin. [29,30]

EUPHORBIA IPECACUANHA: Root of American ipecac, *Euphorbia ipecacuanha*. Emetic and cathartic; also used as a blister. [29,30]

EUPHORBIUM: Resinous gum from several *Euphorbia* spp. Potent emetic, cathartic, and vesicant, but used chiefly only as an errhine. [15,29]

EUPHRASIA: Leaves of eye-bright, *Euphrasia officinalis*. Internal and external ophthalmic remedy. [15]

Exipotica: Remedies that aid digestion.

Expectorant: A drug that promotes secretion and rejection of mucus and other fluids from the lungs and trachea. Used in, e.g., pneumonia, catarrh, and asthma.

Extergentia: Detergent remedies that clean and dry suppurating wounds and sores.

EYE-BRIGHT: See EUPHRASIA.

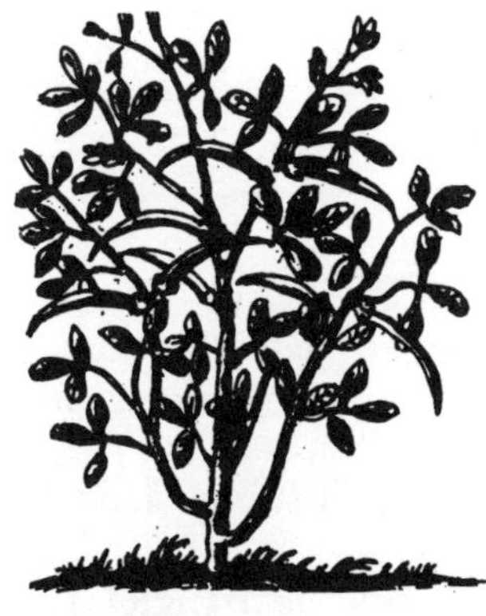

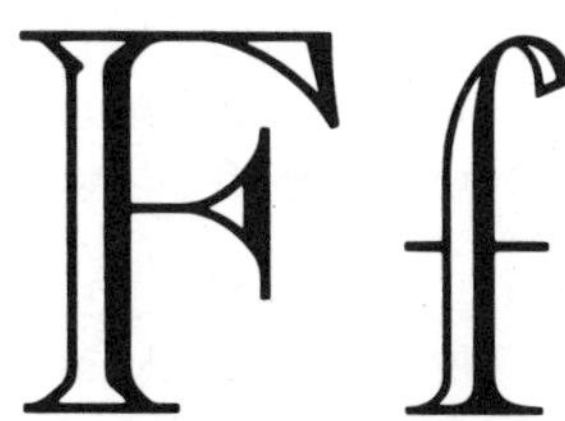

Foenum graecum

FABA: Broad beans, *Vicia faba*. A flatulent but nutritious food. [15]

FAEX VINI: Same as CREAM OF TARTAR.

FARFARA: Same as TUSSILAGO.

FARINA: Wheat. Used in poultices for skin inflammations, and for the nutritive value of its gluten content.

FARINA VIRGINEA: A tooth powder.

FEATHERFEW: See MATRICARIA.

Febrifuge: A drug that removes fever; essentially, an Antiphlogistic, q.v.

FELIX: See FILIX.

FENNEL, SWEET: See FOENICULUM DULCE.

FENUGREEK: Seeds of *Trigonella foenum-graecum*. Aromatic, aphrodisiac, and sometimes used for hemorrhoids and emollient cataplasms. [2]

FERMENTI, CATAPLASMA: "Fermenting poultice," made with flour and yeast. [23]

FERNS: See FILIX, LYCOPERDON, SCOLOPENDRIUM, and TRICHOMANES.

FERRI COMPOSITA, MISTURA: 1) "Compound mixture of iron," made with MYRRH, LIXIVA, AQUA ROSAE, spirit of NUTMEG, FERRUM VITRIOLATUM (although, paradoxically, it could be omitted), and sugar. Tonic and antihectic. 2) See IRON, COMPOUND MIXTURE OF.

FERRI CUM MYRRHA, PILULE: "Iron and myrrh pill," made with FERRUM VITRIOLATUM, MYRRH, SUBCARBONAS SODAE, and sugar.

FERRI FERROCYANURETUM: Ferric ferrocyanide, Prussian blue. Tonic, febrifuge, and alterative. [29]

FERRI LIMATURA PREPARATA: "Prepared iron filings." Same as FERRI RUBIGO.

FERRI LIMATURA PURIFICATA: "Purified iron filings," collected from a blacksmith shop and purified by attracting them through gauze with a magnet. Used in preparing several iron remedies.

FERRI OXIDUM NIGRUM: Same as FERRI LIMATURA PURIFICATA, after powdering.

FERRI RAMENTA: "Iron filings," same as FERRI LIMATURA PURIFICATA.

FERRI RUBIGO: "Iron rust," red iron oxides, chiefly ferric oxide. Used to stimulate menstruation, especially in patients with chlorosis (now known to have been iron deficiency anemia), as a tonic, and in preparing other FERRUM compounds. [15,46] Also see FERRUM.

FERRI SQUAMAE PURIFICATAE: "Purified iron scales," same as FERRI LIMATURA PURIFICATA.

FERRI, VINUM: Iron filings in wine. [15]

FERRUM: Iron. French apothecary and chemist Nicolas Lémery had found it in the blood in the late 17th century. Astringent and styptic; a tonic stimulant of the circulation; cathartic, diaphoretic, and diuretic; sometimes emetic. The onset of its effect is detectable by black stools. "Iron is the only metal which seems naturally friendly to the animal body." [15]

FERRUM AMMONIATUM (or AMMONIACALE): Ferric chloride. Aperient, antihysteric, and tonic. [15]

FERRUM [RUBRUM] PRAECIPITATUM, TINCTURA: "Tincture of iron rust." Tonic; sometimes given with added ANGUSTURA for stomach pain. Also see FERRI RUBIGO. [1]

FERRUM TARTARISATUM: Iron tartrates. Tonic. [15]

FERRUM VITRIOLATUM: Ferrous sulfate. Astringent,

tonic, diuretic, emmenagogue, and anthelminthic. Side effects include nausea and stomach pain. [1,15,29,30]

FERRUM VITRIOLATUM EXSICCATUM (or USTUM): Heat-dried FERRUM VITRIOLATUM.

FERULA ASAFOETIDA: Same as ASAFOETIDA.

FERULA PERSICA: See SAGAPENUM.

FERULA TINGITANA: See SILPHIUM.

FETID TINCTURE, POWDER, or PILL: Its chief ingredient was ASAFOETIDA.

FEVER-ROOT (or FEVERWORT): See TRIOSTEUM.

FICUS CARICA: Same as CARICA.

FIG: See CARICA.

FIGWORT: See SCROPHULARIA NODOSA.

FILIX [MAS]: Root of male fern, *Dryopteris felix-mas*. Anthelminthic; slightly tonic and astringent. [15,23,29] It is effective treatment for tapeworms; see NOUFFER'S TAPEWORM CURE.

FIOVARENTI, BAUME DE: A tincture of CANELLA, CARYOPHYLLUS AROMATICUS, NUTMEG, ZINGIBER, LAURUS, SUCCINUM, GALBANUM, MYRRH, ALOES, ELEMI, and other aromatics, with added TEREBINTHA VENETA. The original formula, which was somewhat different, was devised about 1650 by Leonardo Fiovarenti, of Bologna, as an antidote to arsenic. The 18th–century formula was used, rarely, for kidney and joint disease. [2]

FIXED AIR: Carbon dioxide. Used chiefly to manufacture SODA WATERS; stimulant, diaphoretic, and diuretic. [30] Also see Antiphlogistic.

FIXED VEGETABLE ALKALI: Same as LIXIVA.

FLAMULA JOVIS: Leaves and flowers of virgin's-bower, *Clematis vitalba*. Acrid vesicant and dangerously potent internal tonic. [15]

FLAVUM, PRAECIPITATUM: "Yellow precipitate," same as HYDRARGYRUS VITRIOLATUS.

FLAVUS, BALSAM: "Yellow balm," same as TURPETH MINERALIS.

FLAX: See LINUM.

FLAX, PURGING: See LINUM CATHARTICUM.

FLAX, TOAD-: See LINARIA.

FLEABANES: See ERIGERON entries.

FLEAWORT: See PSYLLIUM.

FLORES SULPHURIS: "Flowers of sulfur;" see SULPHUR.

FLORUM OMNIUM, AQUA: "Water of all flowers," cow urine. For intestinal disorders; externally, for cutaneous disease.

FLOS CORDIALUM: "Flower of cordials," an elixir of unknown composition said to have extraordinary cordial properties.

FLOWER DE LUCE: See IRIS PSEUDACORUS.

FLOWERS OF SULPHUR: See SULPHUR.

Fluidounce (or Fluiduncia): See Measurement.

Fluidrachm (or Fluidrachma): See Measurement.

FOENICULUM DULCE: Seeds and root of sweet fennel, *Foeniculum vulgare*. An aromatic carminative, resolvent, expectorant, diuretic, and lactagogue. [15,23,29]

FOENUM GRAECUM: Same as FENUGREEK.

FOETIDAE, PILULE: "Stinking pill" made of 19 ingredients. Cathartic.

FOLIAE: Leaves.

Fomentation: 1) A warm medicated decoction applied to the body on flannel, linen, or sponges, or squeezed from a bladder. 2) Some enemas. [12,15]

FONTANA, AQUA: "Spring water," used as a diluent. [1]

FONTICULOS, EMPLASTRUM AD: A Sparadrapum.

Fonticulus: Literally, "little fountain;" jargon for UNGUENTUM CANTHARIDIS. [1]

FORMICAE CUM ACERVO: Literally, "a heap of ants." Distillate containing formic acid made by infusing "a quantity of live and vigorous ants" in water. Discovered in 1670 by S. Fisher, while he was distilling a mass of ants. Aphrodisiac. [15]

FORTIS, AQUA: "Strong water." Same as ACIDUM NITRICUM.

FOSSILE, SAL: Rock salt; see SAL MURIATICUS.

FOTHERGILL'S PILLS: A 19th-century proprietary cathartic made with ALOES, SCAMMONIUM, COLOCYNTHIS, and CROCUS ANTIMONII.

Fotus: An emollient cataplasm.

FOWLER'S SOLUTION: Same as SOLUTIO MINERALIS ARSENICI. Introduced by Dr. Thomas Fowler of Stafford, Shropshire, in 1785. [ref. 4, p. 210].

FOXGLOVE: See DIGITALIS.

FRACASTORII [FULLERI] [SINE MELLE], CONFEC-

TIO: "Confection of Fracastoro [or of Fuller] [without honey]." An antidysenteric confection attributed to the 16th–century Italian physician Girolamo Fracastoro, and reintroduced in the 18th century by Dr. Thomas Fuller of London. [20]

FRAGA: Strawberries, *Fragaria* spp., and their leaves. Refrigerant, weak tonic, diuretic, and cathartic; not nutritious. [15]

FRANKFURT PILL: A cathartic mixture of ALOES and RHEI invented by Dr. Johann Hartmann Beyer of Frankfurt in the early 17th century.

FRANKINCENSE: See OLIBANUM and THUS.

FRASERA CAROLINENSIS (or WALTHERI): See COLUMBA, AMERICAN.

FRAXINELLA: Same as DICTAMNUS ALBUS.

FRAXINUS: Bark and seeds of ash, *Fraxinus excelsior*, and other spp. The bark was considered astringent, and the seeds aperient, but the latter were seldom used. [15]

FRAXINUS ORNUS: Same as GUM MANNA.

FRENCH BOLE: A pale red BOLUS that effervesces slightly with acids.

FRENCH LAVENDER: See STECHAS.

FRIAR'S BALSAM: A liniment much like TINCTURA BENZOINI COMPOSITA.

Friction: A poultice designed to chafe and redden the skin, to simulate its circulation. [1]

FRIER'S DROPS: A mixture of CALOMEL, ANTIMONIUM, GUIAC, BALSAM OF PERU, HEMLOCK, oil of SASSAFRAS, CREAM OF TARTAR (?), GUM ARABIC, and SPIRITUS VINI; patented by Robert Grubb in 1777 and advertised as a cure for venereal disease, scurvy, rheumatism, and urinary tract disorders. [13]

FROBENIUS, LIQUEUR DE: Same as AETHER VITRIOLICUS, which a 16th-century alchemist, Wilhelmus Godofredus Frobenius, called after himself.

Frontal: A headache remedy to be applied to the forehead.

FUGA DAEMONUM: "Flight of demons," so-called because hanging it in a window on St. John's Day, 27 December, virtually always kept evil spirits away. Same as HYPERICUM.

FULIGO LIGNI: "Wood soot." Antihysteric. [15]

FULMINANS, PULVIS: "Fulminating powder," made of NITER, SAL TARTARI, and SULPHUR, which, when fused in fire, makes a loud noise. Also see PULVIS TORMENTORIUS.

FUMARIA: Leaves of fumitory, *Fumaria officinalis*. Tonic for bowels; diuretic, cathartic, diaphoretic, and antiscorbutic; emmenagogue; anthelminthic; blood purifier. [15]

FUMITORY: See FUMARIA.

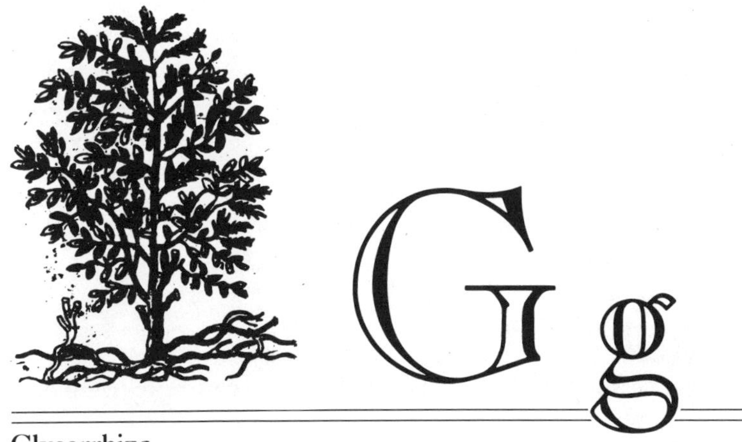

Glycerrhiza

Galactopoetica: Lactagogues.

GALANGA MINOR: Root of galingale genera *Kaempferia* and *Alpinia* imported from East Indies (not to be confused with "English galingale," *Cyperus longa*). Stomachic bitter. [2,6,15]

GALBANUM: Gum resin of *Ferula galbaniflua*. Deobstruent, antihysteric, antispasmodic, stimulant, emmenagogue, and expectorant. [15,29,30] Applied externally as a discutient and to promote suppuration. [23]

GALENA: Lead ore, chiefly lead sulfide.

GALENE: A version of MITHRIDATE.

GALE'S SPA ELIXIR: A tonic medicine containing FERRUM patented in 1782.

GALINGALE: See GALANGA MINOR.

GALLA: Gall nuts, a reaction of tree bark tissues to the secretions of larvae of gall wasps (chiefly *Cynips quercifolii*) as they emerge from eggs laid in oriental oak (*Quercus cerris*) or dyer's oak, *Q. infectoria*. Strong astringent for topical use; occasionally used internally as a tonic. [2,15,23,29] Contains tannins that precipitate proteins and have, therefore, been used as antidiarrheals.

GALLIA MOSCHATA: "French musk," a cordial and stimulant troche made of MOSCHUS, SUCCINUM, and ALOES.

GALLICUS, BOLUS: Same as FRENCH BOLUS.

GALL NUTS: See GALLA.

Gallon: See Measurement.

GAMBOGE or GAMBOGIA: Gum resin of *Garcinia hanburii.* Introduced to Europe from southeast Asia by French physician Charles de Lécluse in 1603, and promoted in England by the East India Company from 1615. Dangerously potent emetic and cathartic; anthelminthic. [15,23,29,30]

GAMBOGIAE COMPOSITAE, PILULE: "Compound gamboge pill," made with GAMBOGE, ALOES, CINNAMOMUM, and soap. Cathartic. [23]

GARCINIA: See GAMBOGE.

Gargar[isma]: A gargle.

GARGET: Same as PHYTOLACCA DECANDRA.

Gargle: A medicated throat remedy, often with astringent and antiseptic properties.

GARLIC: Extract of garlic, *Allium sativum.* Administered orally as a tonic, diaphoretic, expectorant, diuretic, carminative, and emmenagogue, or applied externally as a rubefacient. Its side effects include headache, flatus, fever, and piles; contraindicated for patients with ileus. The active principle is absorbed through the skin and exhaled through the lungs. [1,15,23,29]

GASCOIGN'S [or GASCOYN'S] POWDER: An expensive preparation of BEZOAR, SUCCINUM, HARTSHORN, CORALLINA, MARGARITAE, and CHELAE CANCER, introduced in the early 17th century.

GAULTHERIA: Leaves of wintergreen, partridge berry, or checkerberry, *Gaultheria procumbens.* Aromatic astringent, antidiarrheal, emmenagogue, and lactagogue, but used chiefly as flavoring. [29,30] Contains salicylic acid, which shares some of the effects of its derivative acetylsalicylic acid (aspirin).

GAUTIER, EMPLASTRUM: A Sparadrapum.

GEMMAE, SAL: Rock salt; see SAL MURIATICUS.

GENISTA: Tops and seeds of various genera of broom (e.g., *Genista* and *Cytisus*). Cathartic; emetic. [15] Produces toxic effects like those of CICUTA.

GENTIAN (or GENTIANA LUTEA) : 1) Root of gentian, *Gentiana lutea.* A tonic but non-astringent bitter for stimulating the appetite, digestion, and circulation; see IN-

FUSUM AMARUM. Side effects include vomiting and catharsis. [1,2,15,23,29] 2) In U.S., sometimes blue gentian, *G. catesbei*, or other spp. with similar properties. [30]

GENTIANAE COMPOSITUM, INFUSUM: "Compound infusion of gentian." Same as INFUSUM AMARUM.

GENTIANAE COMPOSITUM, TINCTURA: "Compound tincture of gentian." Alcohol extract of same ingredients used in INFUSUM AMARA.

GENTIANAE COMPOSITUM, VINUM: "Compound wine of gentian." Same as VINUM AMARUM.

GENTINA: See CURSUTA.

GEOFFROEA [INERMIS]: Bark of cabbage tree, any of several Caribbean palm spp., e.g., *Andira inermis*. Anthelminthic. Its side effects include emesis, catharsis, delirium, and fever. [15,23,29]

GERANIUM MACULATUM: Plant and root of wild geranium, or cranesbill, *Geranium maculatum*. Antiseptic and antidiarrheal astringent. [23.29,30]

GERANIUM OIL: See CAMEL'S HAY.

GERMANDER: See CHAMAEDRYS.

GERMANDER, WATER: See SCORDIUM.

GEUM [RIVALE]: Root of water, or purple, avens, also called chocolate root, *Geum rivale*. Tonic, and a potent astringent. [29]

GEUM URBANUM: Same as CARYOPHYLLATA.

GILEAD, BALM OF: 1) In Europe, sap of *Commiphora opobalsamum* or *Amyris gileadensis*. Because it was difficult to procure from Ottoman merchants, it was replaced in general medical usage by CANADA and COPAIVA BALSAMS. [15] 2) In U.S., sometimes Balm of Gilead poplar, *Populus balsamifera*, with similar properties. Also see CARPOBALSAMUM and SOLOMON'S CORDIAL BALM OF GILEAD. The identity of the biblical balm of Gilead is disputed.

GILLA THEOPHRASTI (or VITRIOLI): Same as ZINCUM VITRIOLATUM. Emetic.

GILLENIA: Root of bowman's root, *Gillenia trifoliata*, or American ipecac, *G. stipulata*; both were often called Indian physic. Mild emetic and tonic, and sometimes cathartic. [29,30]

Gilva, Emplastra: Honey-colored plasters.

GINGER: see ZINGIBER.

GINGER, WILD: See ASARUM, def. no. 2.

GINGIVALE, ELECTUARIUM: "Gingival electuary," made

with MYRRH, CREAM OF TARTAR, COCHINEAL, CARYOPHYLLUS, and honey. For sore gums. [15]

GINSENG: Root of *Panax quinquefolius* (from North America) or, less often, *P. schinseng* (from China). Medical applications uncertain, but probably tonic. [15] Regarded as medically useless in America. [29; see Ronald K. Siegel, "Ginseng Abuse Syndrome," *Journal of the American Medical Association 241* (1979): 1614-1615]

GLADIOLUS: See IRIS PALUSTRIS.

GLASS OF ANTIMONY: Same as ANTIMONIUM VITRIFICATUM.

GLAUBER'S SALT: Same as VITRIOLATED SODA. Introduced by German physician and chemist Johann Rudolph Glauber of Amsterdam about 1650 as a cathartic. [2]

GLAUBER'S SECRET SAL AMMONIAC: Ammonium sulfate. Cathartic.

GLAUBER'S SPIRIT OF NITRE: See NITRE, SPIRIT OF.

GLAUBER'S SPIRIT OF SALT: Same as ACIDUM MURIATICUM.

Glutinoria: Remedies that agglutinate and thicken the blood, and arrest hemorrhage.

Glycea: Mild cathartics.

GLYCERRHIZA [GLABRA]: Root of licorice, *Glycerrhiza glabra*. Gentle demulcent cathartic; expectorant and detergent; neutralizes the constipating effect of OPIUM; also allays thirst. Sometimes included in drug mixtures as a menstruum. [1,2,15, 23,29,30] Still used as a demulcent, mild expectorant, and menstruum.

GLYCERRHIZAE COMPOSITAE, PULVIS: "Compound powder of licorice," invented in the 1790s by Ernst Gottfried Kurella of Berlin. A cathartic based on GLYCERRHIZA.

Glyster: An enema, usually administered with a metal syringe, but sometimes squeezed from an animal bladder. [12] Also see ENEMA, DOMESTIC.

GODDARD'S DROPS: A proprietary version of SPIRITUS AMMONIAE AROMATICUS. Probably invented by Dr. William Goddard of London in the mid-17th century, it was originally an oil extracted from human bones; SPIRIT OF NITER and SPIRITUS VINOSUS were added later. Promoted as a panacea. [13]

GODFREY'S CORDIAL: Invented by Ambroise Godfrey of London about 1660, or by Thomas Godfrey of Hertfordshire, and first marketed there by John Fisher, "Physician and Chymist," in 1721. Its chief ingredient was OPIUM; later versions also included SASSAFRAS. [14]

GOLDEN DROPS OF GENERAL LA MOTHE: Tincture of perchloride of iron and ether promoted in the 18th century. [13]

GOLDEN ROD (or GOLDEN ROOT): 1) In Europe, VIRGA AUREA. 2) In U.S., SOLIDAGO.

GOLDEN SEAL: *Hydrastis canadensis.* Introduced from North American Indian usage in the late 18th century. Tonic, vulnerary, escharotic, laxative, antidyspeptic, febrifuge, cholagogue, and for cancer and snake bite. [See Christopher Hobbs, "Golden Seal in Early American Botany," *Pharmacy in History 32* (1990): 79-82.] Contains an alkaloid that has been used as a heart stimulant, although it is toxic to the central nervous system.

GOLDEN SULPHURET: Sulfides of ANTIMONIUM with SULPHUR.

GOLDEN SULPHUR OF ANTIMONY: Same as SULPHUR ANTIMONII PRAECIPITATUM.

Goldsmiths' Weights: See Measurement.

GOLDTHREAD: See NIGELLA.

GOULARD'S EXTRACT OF SATURN: CERUSSA ACETATA (actually, lead subacetate) in brandy and water, invented by French surgeon Thomas Goulard of Montpellier about 1760. Used in plasters, especially for superficial "cancers." [2,13,15].

Grain: Unit of weight; see Measurement.

GRAINS OF PARADISE: 1) GRANA PARADISI. 2) Same as CARDAMOMUM MINUS

GRAMEN: Roots of quick-grass, *Triticum repens.* Aperient and blood purifier. [15]

Grana: Grain weights; see Measurement.

GRANA ANGELICA: See ANDERSON'S SCOTS PILLS.

GRANA PARADISI: Fruits of grains of paradise, or Guinea grains, from *Amomum melegueta* or *Aframomum* spp. Carminative. [15]

GRANATA MALUS, or GRANATUM: Flowers, or rind of fruit, of pomegranate, *Punica granatum.* Cooling cathartic; astringent antidiarrheal; anthelminthic. [15,29,30]

GRAPES: See UVA PASSA, VINUM, and VITIS.

GRATIA DEI: "Thanks be to God," a vulnerary plaster resembling one made with BETONICA.

GRATIOLA: Leaves of hedge hyssop, *Gratiola officinalis*. Strong cathartic. [15]

GREGORY'S POWDER: A mixture of RHEI and MAGNESIA USTA devised by Dr. James Gregory of Edinburgh in the late 18th century.

GRIFFITH'S MIXTURE: Essentially, same as PILULE FERRI CUM MYRRHA.

GROUNDPINE: See CHAMAEPITHYS.

GROUNDSEL: *Senecio vulgaris*. Refrigerant; antiscorbutic. The word groundsel means, in Old English, "to swallow pus."

Gtt.: Abbreviation for Gutta (drops); see Measurement.

GUALTERI, TELA: See TELA GUALTERI.

GUIAC, GUIAIAC, or GUAIACUM [OFFICINALE]: Resin and wood of lignum vitae, *Guaiacum officinale*, or *G. sanctum*. Introduced from Hispaniola to Europe in 1508, and first promoted as an antivenereal in 1519. Stimulant diaphoretic, diuretic, and cathartic; used especially in treating syphilis. [1,2,12,15,23,29,30; also see Paul A. Russell, "Syphilis, God's Scourge or Nature's Vengeance?," *Archiv für Reformationgeschichte 80* (1989): 286-307.] Two derivatives, guaiacol and guaifenesin, are still used as expectorants, and the guaiac test is used to detect small amounts of blood in the stool.

GUIACI COMPOSITUM, DECOCTUM: Made with GUIAC, SASSAFRAS, GLYCERRHIZA, and UVA PASSA. For cutaneous manifestations of "foulness of the blood and juices," to combat excessive phlegm, and to counteract excessive cathartic reactions to mercury or antimony. [15]

GUILANDINA MORINGA: See NEPHRITICUM LIGNUM.

GUINEA GRAINS: See GRANA PARADISI.

GUMMOSA, PILULE: A "gum-pill" made with MYRRH and OPOPANAX.

GUM PILL: Same as PILULE ASAFOETIDAE COMPOSITAE.

Gutta: Drops; see Measurement.

GUTTETAM, PULVIS AD: Powder of PAEONIA, VALERIAN, DICTAMNUS ALBUS, HARTSHORN, MOTHER-OF-PEARL, and VISCUS. Antiepileptic ("gutteta" was a Languedoc word for epilepsy); antihysteric; for vertigo; and anodyne.

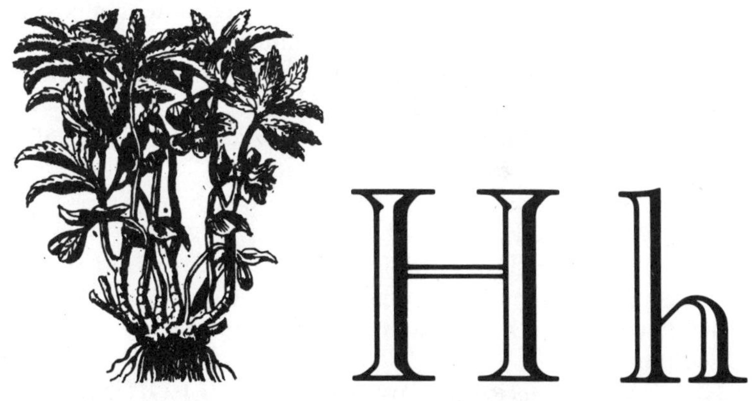

Helleborus niger

HAARLEM DROPS: Same as DUTCH DROPS.

HAEMATOXYLUM [CAMPECHIANUM]: Logwood, *Haematoxylon campechianum*. A distinctive red dye from South America, it was introduced to medicine by 1746. Mild non-irritating astringent, tonic, and antidiarrheal. [1,15,23,29,30; also see John J. Gurecki, "The History of Hematoxylin," *Laboratory Medicine 15* (1984): 423-425] Now used for staining microscopic tissue sections.

HAEMORRHOIDALE, UNGUENTUM: "Hemorrhoid ointment" made of SATURNINE OINTMENT, HYOSCYAMUS, CAMPHOR, and CROCUS. Emollient and anodyne. [15]

HALY [ABBAS], POWDER OF: Made with poppy seeds (possibly from PAPAVER SOMNIFERUM), GUM ARABIC, GLYCERRHIZA, SPODIUM, and AMYLUM. Named for Haly ben Abbas, a 10th-century Persian medical encyclopedist. Antitussive.

HAMAMELIS VIRGINIANA: Bark of witch hazel, *Hamamelis virginiana*. Astringent. [23]

HARDHACK: See SPIRAEA TOMENTOSA.

HARTSHORN: 1) Calcium phosphates extracted from stag

horns. General tonic, a property inferred from the annual renewal of horns; diaphoretic, febrifuge; alexipharmic; sedative, antispasmodic, antiepileptic, nervine, rubefacient, absorbent, antacid, and vermifuge; sometimes used in rickets. [1,2,15,23] 2) Probably usually same as AQUA AMMONIAE. 3) Now defined as ammonium carbonate, a mixture of ammonium bicarbonate and ammonium carbamate in water, producing 30–34% ammonia and 45% carbon dioxide.

Haustus: A medicinal draught.

HAUSTUS CATHARTICUS: "Cathartic draught," usually a mixture of several active ingredients.

HAZELWORT: See ASARUM.

HEAL-ALL: See PRUNELLA.

HEALTH, ELIXIR OF: Same as ELIXIR SALUTIS.

HEAT: Warm compresses applied to the abdomen, or a bath heated above 84°F. to relax the stomach to prevent repeated vomiting. [1]

HEDEOMA: American pennyroyal; see PULEGIUM.

HEDERA ARBOREA: Leaves and resin of common ivy, *Hedera helix*. An internal tonic for children; an external dressing used to keep therapeutic blisters running or as a depilatory. The berries are said to be diaphoretic and alexipharmic. [15]

HEDERA TERRESTRIS: Leaves of ground ivy, *Glechoma hederacea*. Tonic, aperient, expectorant, and a blood purifier. [15]

Hedychroum: A saffron-colored alexipharmic troche.

Hedysmata: Aromatic unguents.

HELLEBORASTER: Leaves of bear's foot, *Helleborus foetidus* (sometimes, erroneously, called black hellebore, which is HELLEBORUS NIGER, q.v.). An anthelminthic especially suitable for children. [15]

HELLEBORE, AMERICAN: See VERATRUM VIRIDE.

HELLEBORUS ALBUS: Same as VERATRUM ALBUM; also see VERATRUM VIRIDE.

HELLEBORUS NIGER: Roots of black hellebore or Christmas rose, *Helleborus niger* (not related to HELLEBORUS ALBUS). A drastic cathartic with emmenagogue and alterative properties. Side effects include vomiting, vertigo, abdominal cramps, convulsions, and death. [15,23,29] Contains 0.2–0.5% of the antimuscarinic alkaloid hyoscyamine, as well as cardiotoxic digitalis–like glycosides and gastro–intestinal irritant saponins.

HEL[L]ENIUM: Same as ENULA CAMPANA.

HELVETII, PULVIS STYPTICUS: See STYPTICUS, PULVIS.

Hemagogus: An emmenagogue, or a drug that stimulates the expulsion of lochia after childbirth.

HEMATITE[S]: A very hard iron ore, sometimes called bloodstone (but not what is now called by that name), composed chiefly of Fe_2O_3. Uses same as those of FERRUM. [15]

HEMLOCK, EMPLASTRUM: Resin of *Pinus balsamea*. Used internally as a tonic, diuretic, and cathartic; externally, as a discutient. [1,2]

HEMLOCK, OIL OF: An extract of BALSAMUM CANADENSE. Abortifacient. [29]

HEMLOCK, POISON: See CICUTA.

HEMLOCK, WATER: See CICUTA and OENANTHE.

HEMP: See CANNABIS.

HEMP AGRIMONY: See EUPATORIUM.

HEMP, INDIAN: See APOCYNUM CANNABINUM.

HENBANE [BLACK]: Same as HYOSCYAMUS.

HENNA: See ALKANET.

Hepar: A chemical with the color of liver.

HEPAR ANTIMONII: Same as ANTIMONII, CROCUS.

HEPAR SULPHURIS: Thought to be same as KALI SULPHURATUM. However, now recognized as a mixture of potassium trisulfide and potassium thiosulfate.

HEPATICA: Leaves of liverwort, or round-lobed hepatica, *Hepatica americana*. Mild demulcent tonic and astringent; questionably diuretic and deobstruent. [29]

HEPATIC ALOES: See ALOES.

HERACLEUM [SPHONDYLIUM]: Root of the European cow-parsnip or masterwort, *Heracleum sphondylium* (or the American spp., *H. lanatum*). Antiepileptic; carminative; rubefacient. [23,29,30]

HERBA BRITTANICA: See HYDROLAPATHUM.

HERBA REGINA: "Herb of the Queen," because it cured Queen Catherine de Medicis of migraine headaches in the late 16th century. Same as NICOTIANA.

HERB BENNET: See CARYOPHYLLATA.

HERB CHRISTOPHER: See ACTEA SPICATA.

HERB MERCURY: See MERCURIALIS.

HERMODACTYLUS: "Finger of Hercules." 1) Root of hermodactyl, *Iris tuberosa*. Cathartic. [15] 2) Sometimes, same as COLCHICUM.

HERNIAM, EMPLASTRUM AD: "Hernia plaster." An early precursor formulation of EMPLASTRUM THURIS COMPOSITUM.

Hetica: Epispastics.

HEUCHERA: Rhizome of alumroot, *Heuchera americana*. Potent astringent for external application. [29,30]

HIBISCUS: See ABELMOSCHUS.

HIERA LOGADII: A complex mixture for treating melancholy, vertigo, convulsions, and other afflictions of the brain.

HIERA PACHII: A purging confection.

HIERA PICRA: "Holy Bitters," a tincture of ALOES and CANELLA; also the basis of VINUM ALOES. Cathartic. [2,15]

HIERA SIMPLE: Same as HIERA PICRA.

HIPPOCASTANUM: Powdered fruit of horse chestnut, *Aesculus hippocastanum*. Astringent tonic. Used as an errhine for ophthalmic disorders; the bark is sometimes used for intermittent fevers because its bitterness resembles that of CINCHONA. [15,23]

HIPPOCONDRIAL INFUSION: One to be applied to the hypochondrial area, in the manner of an ANTIHYSTERIC PLASTER. [2]

HIRUDO [MEDICINALIS]: Medicinal leech; see BLEEDING.

HIRUNDINUM, OLEUM: "Oil of swallows," *Hirundo* spp., made with whole swallows and 13 other ingredients.

HOFFMANN'S ANODYNE LIQUOR: A mixture of AETHER VITRIOLICUS and alcohol.

HOFFMANN'S BALSAM OF LIFE: A tincture of BALSAM OF PERU and several aromatics devised in the early 18th century by Dr. Friedrich Hoffmann of Halle. Vulnerary liniment.

HOFFMAN'S DROPS: Nearly same as HOFFMAN'S ANODYNE LIQUOR.

HOFFMAN'S [VISCERAL] ELIXIR: Mixture of GENTIANA, ABSINTHUM, MELLILOT, CASCARILLA, CORTEX AURANTIUM, and CINNAMOMUM. Devised by Dr. Friedrich Hoffmann of Halle.

HOLSATICA, PANACEA: See PANACEA HOLSATICA.

HOLY THISTLE: Same as CARDUUS BENEDICTUS.

HOMBERG'S NARCOTIC SALT OF VITRIOL: A complex preparation of FERRUM VITRIOLATUM and

BORAX, devised in the early 18th century by Dutch chemist Dr. Willem Homberg of Paris.

HONEY: Aperient, detergent, and expectorant. [2,15,23; also see ref. 8, pp. 68-71]

HOOPER'S [FEMALE] PILLS: Patented in 1743 by Dr. John Hooper of Reading, England, as the "best purging stomatik and anti-hysteric" remedy, and later promoted as a tonic cathartic and emmenagogue. Its chief ingredient was ALOES, but by the 19th century FERRUM VITRIOLATUM, MYRRH, and CANELLA had been added. [14]

HOP: See LUPULUS.

HORDEI COMPOSITUM, DECOCTUM: "Compound decoction of barley." Made with HORDEUM, CARICA, GLYCERRHIZA, and UVA PASSA. A nourishing diluent for febrile patients. [15]

HORDEUM [DISTICHON]: Barley, *Hordeum distichon.* Usually, for nourishment and as a refrigerant, but also a demulcent pectoral. [1,2,15,23,29]

HORDEUM PERLATUM: "Pearl barley," polished seeds of HORDEUM.

HOREHOUND, WATER: See LYCOPUS.

HOREHOUND, WHITE: See MARRUBIUM.

HOREHOUND, WILD: See EUPATORIUM PILOSUM.

Horetica: Digestives (in sense of def. no. 1), and appetite stimulants.

HORMINUM SATIVUM: Leaves and seeds of clary, *Salvia sclarea* (and perhaps other spp.). Antihysteric and carminative. [15]

HORSE CHESTNUT: See HIPPOCASTANUM.

HORSE RADISH: See RHAPHANUS RUSTICANUS.

HORSEMINT: See MONARDA.

HORSEWEED: See ERIGERON CANADENSE.

HOUND'S TONGUE: See CYNOGLOSSUS.

HOY'S SALT: Introduced by a Dr. Hoy in the early 18th century as a cheap manufactured form of Epsom salt. Same as MAGNESIA VITRIOLATA.

Humectant: A moistening agent or diluent.

HUMULUS LUPULUS: Same as LUPULUS.

HUNGARY [QUEEN OF] WATER: ROSEMARINUS distilled in wine. Attributed to a legendary formula invented in 1235 by Queen Elizabeth of Hungary. Antispasmodic. [2,13]

HUSSON, EAU MEDICINALE D': A late 18th-century

British proprietary preparation (mysteriously named for a French army officer) of COLCHICUM (but perhaps HELLEBORUS ALBUS). For gout. [13,23]

HUXHAM'S TINCTURE: A mixture of CINCHONA, CORTEX AURANTIUM, SERPENTINA, COCHINEAL, and CROCUS in wine, introduced in the 1750s by Dr. John Huxham of Plymouth, England. Astringent, stomachic, and corroborant in low doses; administered for intermittent fevers at very high doses, but seldom used for that purpose because such doses induce stomach pain. [2,15,20; John Huxham, *An Essay on Fevers* (1757; rprt. ed. Canton, Mass.: Science History Publications, 1988), esp. p. 65].

Hydragogue: A drug that removes excess water via the large intestine.

HYDRARGYRI, EMPLASTRUM: Mercurial plaster made with OL OLIVA, TEREBINTHA, HYDRARGYRUS PURIFICATUS, and CERUSSA ACETATA. Resolvent and discutient; antivenereal. [15]

HYDRARGYRI (sometimes, FORTIUS [strong] or MITIUS [weak] was specified), UNGUENTUM: A mercurial ointment used not for its topical action but to introduce mercury into the circulation through the skin, rather than via the customary oral route. [15]

HYDRARGYRI SUBMURIAS: Same as CALOMEL.

HYDRARGYROSI MURIATI MITIS, PILULE: Pill made of CALOMEL, VITRIOL ANTIMONIUM, and CONSERVE OF ROSES. Cathartic. [1,15]

HYDRARGYRUS: Mercury, administered in many forms (e.g., CALOMEL, HYDRARGYRUS MURIATUS CORROSIVUS, and HYDRARGYRUS PRAECIPITATUS CINEREUS). Although it may have entered general medical practice as early as 1140, it was introduced for the treatment of syphilis in 1497, by Caspar Torella. By the 18th century it was employed as a cathartic, diuretic, diaphoretic, and sialagogue (and sometimes emetic), to stimulate secretions and the circulation in order to promote absorption and removal of "morbific matter" from sites of disease. Because it was "the most general evacuant we possess," it was widely used in the general treatment of many fevers, as a vermifuge, and especially as a "specific" in syphilis, in which mercury was thought to prevent the causative "virus" (i.e., poison) from acting, by expelling it from the body. Salivation ("ptyalism"), accompanied by a metallic taste, was a predictable side effect of all mercurial drugs, and was, therefore, often monitored as a guide to dose adjustments. [1,2,15,23,29,30; also see Paul A. Russell, "Syphilis, God's Scourge or Nature's Vengeance?," *Archiv für Reformationgeschichte 80* (1989): 286-307] Although mercury does kill syphilis organisms upon contact in the test tube, it is not a dependable treatment for syphilis in either animals or human patients. It seems likely that mercury may only inhibit the organisms' growth sufficiently to permit the body's natural defenses to complete their eradication [ref. 33, 1st ed., pp. 986-987].

HYDRARGYRUS ALKALISATUS: Nearly same as HYDRARGYRUS CUM CRETA.

HYDRARGYRUS CALCINATUS: Same as HYDRARGYRUS PRAECIPITATUS.

HYDRARGYRUS CUM CRETA: HYDRARGYRUS [PURIFICATUS] (37-39%) mixed with CRETA. Weak alterative. [15]

HYDRARGYRUS CUM SULFURE: Same as HYDRARGYRUS SULPHURATUS NIGER.

HYDRARGYRUS MURIATUS CORROSIVUS: Corrosive sublimate, or mercuric chloride, $HgCl_2$, introduced for the treatment of syphilis by Dr. Antonio Nuñez Ribero in 1750. Usually applied topically to cutaneous inflammations, or ingested, after dilution, to facilitate the excretion, through feces, urine, and sweat, of contagious factors in patients with, e.g., venereal disease. Regarded as a highy dangerous and potentially fatal drug, it was sometimes administered in a formulation containing SAL AMMONIACUS, ALTHAEA, and HONEY, as well as alone. [1,2,15,23,30]

HYDRARGYRUS MURIATUS MITIS (or PRAECIPITATUS): Same as CALOMEL.

HYDRARGYRUS NITRATUS RUBER: Red mercuric nitrate. A possible alternative to CALOMEL, but used chiefly as a topical escharotic. [23,30]

HYDRARGYRUS OXYMURIAS: Same as HYDRARGYRUS MURIATUS CORROSIVUS.

HYDRARGYRUS PRAECIPITATUS [CINEREUS]: Mercuric oxide. Antisyphilitic; diaphoretic, alterative, cathartic, and emetic, as the dose increases. [1,15,23]

HYDRARGYRUS PURIFICATUS: Elemental MERCURY.

HYDRARGYRUS SULPHURATUS NIGER: Black mercuric sulfide. Although assumed to share the effects of CAL-

OMEL and other mercurials, it was generally thought to be ineffective. [15,23]

HYDRARGYRUS SULPHURATUS RUBER: Red mercuric sulfide, sometimes called "artificial cinnabar" (cf. CINNABAR) or vermilion. Used occasionally in fumigations for syphilitic ulcers, but generally thought to be ineffective. [15,23]

HYDRARGYRUS VITRIOLATUS [FLAVUS]: Mercuric subsulfate, $HgSO_4 \cdot 2H_2O$. Strongest of all mercurial emetics, especially in venereal disease; errhine and diaphoretic; also applied to skin sores and itch. [15,23]

HYDRASTIS: See GOLDEN SEAL.

HYDROCRITHE: "Barley water." Same as AQUA HORDEUM.

HYDROLAPATHUM: Roots of water dock, *Rumex aquaticus* and other spp. Cathartic; used in ointments and cataplasms for scorbutic and other cutaneous conditions, and in mouth washes. Once thought to be an ancient scurvy remedy called Herba Britannica. [15,23]

Hydromel: HONEY in water.

Hydrosaccharum: 1) Simple sugar. 2) A JULAP.

HYDRO-SULPHURETUM AMMONIAE: Probably ammonium sulfide. A sedative that produces vertigo, drowsiness, vomiting, and bradycardia. Used in diabetes to reduce "the morbid appetite and increased action of the stomach." [23]

HYOSCYAMUS [NIGER]: Leaves, roots, and seeds of black henbane, *Hyoscyamus niger*. Introduced by Dr. Anton Störck of Vienna in 1762. Used as a sedative, narcotic, antispasmodic, and anodyne. Like OPIUM, "its influence is very much diminished by habit." Side effects include delirium, mydriasis, weak fluttering pulse, convulsions, diaphoresis, sedation, pustules, vomiting, colic, diarrhea, and diuresis; also produces vertigo, headache, stupor, and analgesia without constipation (the latter unlike OPIUM), and even death. Also used in plasters. [1,15,23,29] Now known to contain atropine-like alkaloids, including scopolamine and hyoscine, which were isolated by Philipp Lorenz Geiger and Germain Henri Hess of Heidelberg in 1833 (also see BELLADONNA). Although scopolamine was said to produce a modest degree of tolerance until the 1960s, its effects are not now thought to be "diminished by habit."

HYPERICUM: Flowers of St. John's wort, *Hypericum per-*

foratum or other spp. Tonic, diuretic, vulnerary, antihysteric, and anthelminthic. [15] Also see FUGA DAEMONUM.

Hypnotica: Remedies that induce sleep.

Hypoglotis, Pilule: A pill for sublingual administration.

Hypolata: Remedies that empty the kidneys, bladder, and liver.

HYSSOP, HEDGE: See GRATIOLA.

HYSSOPUS [OFFICINALIS]: Leaves of garden hyssop, *Hyssopus officinalis*. Expectorant, antitussive, pectoral, and carminative. [15,23]

HYSTERIC JULEP WITH MUSK [OF BATE]: Same as MISTURA MOSCHATA, but made with ORANGE-flower water instead of ROSE-water. [15]

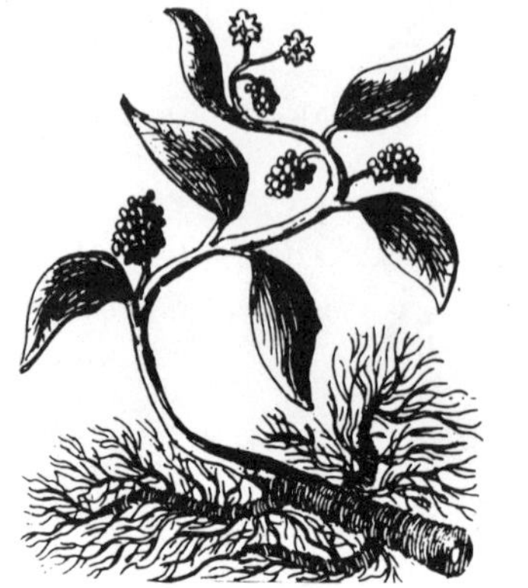

I i

Ipecacuanha

ICELAND MOSS: See LICHEN.

ICHTHYOCOLLA: Isinglass, or fish glue, extracted from skin of sturgeons (Acipenseridae) and other fish, but sometimes gelatin was meant. Demulcent and emollient. Used in plasters, and as nourishment. [2,23,29] N.B.: Modern isinglass has a very different definition.

ILEX: See PRINOS.

IMPERATORIA: Root of masterwort, probably *Peucedanum* (*Imperatoria*) *osthruthium*, but other genera shared the same common name (see, e.g., HERACLEUM). Aromatic. [15]

IMPERIALIS, PILULE: "Imperial pill," made with ALOES, RHEI, AGARICUS, SENNA, CINNAMOMUM, ZINGIBER, MOSCHATA, CARYOPHYLLUS AROMATICUS, NARDUS INDICA, MASTICHE, and VIOLA. Cathartic.

Imperial Measures: See Measurement.

Incider: A medicine containing sharp particles that cut offending humors, rendering them less viscous and, therefore, less likely to form obstructions.

Incitant: A stimulant.

Incrassating drug: One that condenses, or thickens, body fluids.

INDIAN HEMP: See APOCYNUM CANNABINUM.

INDIAN NARD: See NARDUS INDICA.

INDIAN PHYSIC: See GILLENIA, and entries for SPIRAEA.

INDIAN PINKROOT: See SPIGELIA.

INDIAN POKE: See HELLEBORUS ALBUS and VERATRUM VIRIDE.

INDIAN TOBACCO: See LOBELIA INFLATA.

INDIAN TURNIP: See ARUM TRIPHYLLUM.

INDIA, PRIDE OF: Same as MELIA AZEDARACH.

INDICA LOPEZIANA, RADIX: Root of Lopez tree (named for Portuguese explorer Juan Lopez Pigneiro), *Toddalia aculeata*, related to ARALIA SPINOSA. Introduced to Europe by Dr. Francesco Redi of Arezzo in 1671, and to European medicine by Dr. Hieronymus David Gaub of Leyden in 1771. Slightly astringent antidiarrheal.

INDIGO: Extract of *Indigofera tinctoria*. Tonic, febrifuge, antispasmodic, and emmenagogue. In 1826, Otto Unverdorben extracted from indigo an alkaline oil that, in 1840, Carl Julius Fritzsche named aniline (because the Spanish word for indigo is *anil*). Aniline drugs (and dyes) were being synthesized by the late 19th century.

INDIGO, WILD: See SOPHORA TINCTORIA.

INFANTUM, PULVIS: "Baby powder." Made of MAGNESIA ALBA and RHEI. Antacid and antidiarrheal for infants. [15]

Infusion: An extract obtained by pouring freshly boiled water over the raw ingredient(s).

Injection: A drug to be inserted into a natural orifice of the body, usually the rectum, and sometimes the urethra or vagina (but never a vein).

Insiccating drug: One that dries the body (e.g., a diuretic).

Inspissated juice: One that has been concentrated by evaporation over heat. Also see Rob.

INULA [HELENIUM]: Same as ENULA CAMPANA.

IODINE: Discovered in seaweed ashes in 1811 by French chemist Bernard Courtois. First used to treat goiter by Dr. Charles Coindet, Sr., of Geneva, in 1820, and first promoted for treating wounds by Dr. John Davies of Hertford in 1839. General stimulant, especially of the digestive organs and other absorbent tissues, and of the lymph glands (in, e.g., scrofula); corrosive, irritant, desiccant, tonic, diuretic, diaphoretic, and emmenagogue. Side effects include ptyalism, skin eruptions, restlessness, palpitations, abdominal pain, vomiting, diarrhea, and death, as dose increases. [29] Now used chiefly as a disinfectant.

IPECAC, or IPECACUANHA: Root of *Cephaelis ipecacuanha*. Introduced to European medicine in the 1640s by Dutch physician Wilhelm Piso and promoted in the early 18th century by his countryman, J. C. Adrian Helvetius, for the treatment of dysentery. In the early 19th century, the gray, or Peruvian, form was preferred to the brown, or Brazilian, root; a white form was regarded as ineffective. Used primarily as a mild, safe, and dependable emetic, but also, in smaller doses, as a diaphoretic and expectorant. Suitable for the treatment of most fevers, and of OPIUM poisoning. Often administered as DOVER'S POWDER. [1,2,15,23,29,30] Ipecac is still used to make some poison victims vomit the poison and, until recently, it was used as an expectorant. The active alkaloid, emetine, was isolated by French chemist Pierre-Joseph Pelletier and Dr. François Magendie in 1817, and separately introduced into medical practice by Magendie in 1821; introduced as specific therapy for amoebic abscess in 1911, by U.S. Army surgeon Dr. Edward B. Vedder while working in the Philippines.

IPECAC, AMERICAN: See EUPHORBIA IPECACUANHA and GILLENIA.

IPECACUANHAE COMPOSITUS, PULVIS: Same as DOVER'S POWDER.

IPOMOEA TURPETHUM: See TURPETHUM.

IRIS FLORENTINA: Root of *Iris florentina*. Strong cathartic, emetic, and diuretic; applied externally as a rubefacient and irritant. [15,29]

IRISH MOSS: See CHONDRUS.

IRIS PALUSTRIS: Roots of yellow water-flag, *Iris pseudocorus*. Strong cathartic. [15]

IRIS PSEUDACORUS: Root of blue flag, or flower de luce, *Iris versicolor*, *I. prismatica*, and other spp. Cathartic, emetic, and diuretic. [23,29]

IRIS TUBEROSA: See HERMODACTYLUS.

IRIS VERSICOLOR: Same as IRIS PSEUDACORUS.

IRON: See FERRUM.

IRON, COMPOUND MIXTURE OF: 1) Essentially, same as PILULE FERRI CUM MYRRHA. 2) See MISTURA FERRI COMPOSITA.

ISINGLASS: Same as ICHTHYOCOLLA.

ISIS NOBILIS: "Noble Isis [i.e., Venus]." Same as CORALLIUM RUBRUM, def. no. 2, when used as an antivenereal.

IVY: See HEDERA entries.

IVY, POISON: See RHUS entries.

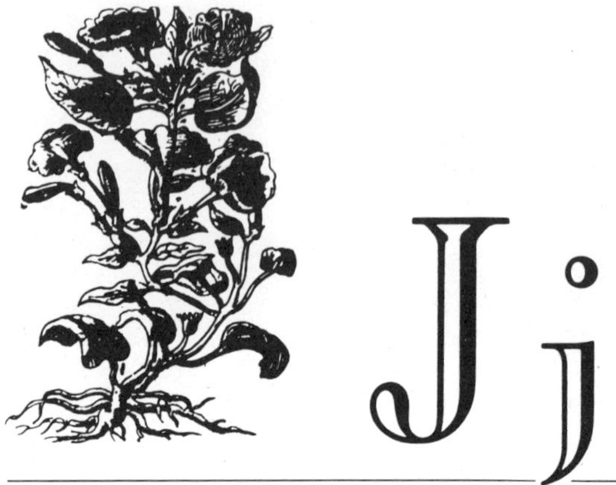

Jalapa

JACK-IN-THE-PULPIT, SMALL: See ARUM TRIPHYLLUM.

JACK-O'LANTERNS: See ALKEKENGI.

JALAP, JALAPA, or JALAPIUM: Powdered root of *Exogonium purga*. Introduced from Mexico to Spanish medicine in 1609. A mild and safe cathartic; diuretic; anthelminthic. [1,15,23,29,30] The active cathartic principle, convolvulin, isolated in 1852-55, irritates the small bowel so as to inhibit the reabsorption of water from the lumen. Still used as a cathartic.

JALAPPAE COMPOSITUS, PULVIS: "Compound powder of jalap," made of JALAP and CREAM OF TARTAR. The latter was thought to potentiate the former, which was, in turn, thought to modulate the refrigerant action of the cream of tartar; the combination was said to "purge the whole system" of morbid matter. [1]

JAMAICA EXTRACT: From the bark of the Florida seagrape, *Coccolobis uviflora*. In the 1790s this drug appeared in the shops of Edinburgh, where it was sold as a dye and, mixed with VALERIAN, as a secret remedy with astringent properties. Twenty years later, resin from the same plant had become the most widely exploited source of GUM KINO. Used—unsuccessfully—as an experimental astringent tonic, and as a substitute for CATECHU. [1]

JAMAICA PEPPER: See PIMENTO.

JAMES'S POWDER: Same as PULVIS ANTIMONIALIS, q.v. One story has it that Dr. Robert James was not awarded a patent when he applied for one in 1760 because the medicine had been in use for 120 years by then, while another version says that James's powder was patented in 1747. [15]

JAMESTOWN WEED: Same as STRAMONIUM.

JAPAN EARTH: Same as CATECHU.

JAPONICA, CONFECTIO: Same as ELECTUARIUM CATECHU.

JAPONICA, TERRA: Same as CATECHU.

JAPONICUM, INFUSUM: Same as CATECHU, INFUSUM.

JASMINUM: Flowers of jasmine, *Jasminum officinalis*. Sometimes recommended for hastening delivery and as an emmenagogue. [15]

JERUSALEM OAK: See BOTRYS.

JESUITS' DROPS: A liniment much like TINCTURA BENZOINI COMPOSITA.

JESUITS' POWDER: Same as CINCHONA, which was brought to Europe by the Jesuits for a time.

JIMSON WEED: "Jamestown weed;" same as STRAMONIUM.

JOVIALE: "Made with Jupiter," i.e., tin; see STANNUM and entries immediately below.

JOVIALE, DIAPHORETICUM: "Diaphonetic of Jupiter," made of STANNUM and ANTIMONIUM CALCINATUM. Antihectic.

JOVIALE, ELECTUARIUM: "Electuary of Jupiter," made of STANNUM, HYDRARGYRUS PURIFICATUS, ABSINTHUM, MENTHA, and OSTREA EDULIS. Anthelminthic. [15]

JOVIS, SAL: "Salt of Jupiter," the nitrate or chloride of STANNUM. Vermifuge.

JUGLANS [CINEREA]: Inner bark and unripe fruit of butternut, or white walnut, *Juglans cinerea*. Weakly anti-inflammatory and emollient. [15] Mild cathartic. [23,29,30]

JUJUBA: Jujubes, fruits of *Zizyphus spina-Christi*. Deobstruent and decongestant. [15]

Julap, or Julep: A sweet aqueous medication, usually with

alterative properties; the word is derived from a Persian word for rose-water. Julep had become an alcoholic beverage in the American south by the 1790s. [Richard Barksdale Harwell, *The Mint Julep* (Charlottesville: University Press of Virginia, 1975)]

JULAP, or JULEP, MUCILAGINOUS: Same as MUCILAGINOUS MIXTURE.

JULAP, or JULEP, SALINE: Frequently, a mixture of LIXIVA, SUCCUS LIMONI, and syrup of RIBES; many similar mixtures were also called julaps, but most were gently diaphoretic and/or diuretic. [1,15]

JULEPUM E MOSCHO: Same as MISTURA MOSCHATA.

JULY-FLOWERS: See CARYOPHYLLUM RUBRUM.

JUNIPERI COMPOSITUS, SPIRITUS: "Compound spirit of juniper," made with JUNIPER berries, CARUM, FOENICULUM DULCE seeds, and alcohol. Diuretic and cordial; used for catarrh, dyspepsia, and oliguria. [1,15]

JUNIPERUS [COMMUNIS]: Berries and tops of juniper, *Juniperus communis* (or *J. sabina*). Carminative, stomachic, intestinal tonic; diaphoretic, diuretic; emmenagogue. Also see SABIN. [1,2,15]

JUNIPERUS, SPIRITUS: In French, *Genièvre*; Anglicized as Geneva, and contracted as gin.

JUNIPERUS VIRGINIANA: Tops of red cedar, *Juniperus virginiana*. Stimulant, emmenagogue, diuretic, and diaphoretic, but less potent than SABIN, *J. sabina*. [29,30]

JUSQUIAMUS: Same as HYOSCYAMUS.

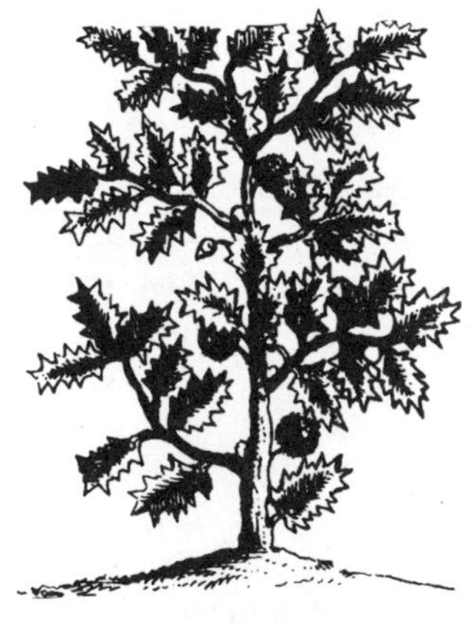

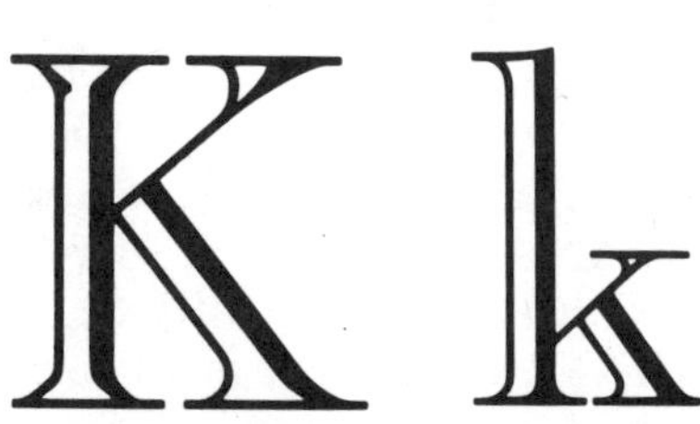

Kermes

KALI [IMPURI]: Same as LIXIVA.

KALI NITRATUM: Same as SAL NITRITI.

KALI SULPHURATUM (or KALI VITRIOLATUM): Potassium sulfate. Administered internally as a mild cathartic and diaphoretic with a relatively long duration of action, and as an antidote to mineral poisons, e.g., mercury, because many metals form insoluble precipitates with sulfur. Applied topically for skin disease. [1]

KALIUM ACETICUM: Same as POTASSAE, ACETIS.

KALMIA ANGUSTIFOLIA: Leaves of lambkill, *Kalmia angustifolia*. Effects like those of KALMIA LATIFOLIA. Contains the poisonous principle grayantoxoin I (for which see RHODODENDRON). [23]

KALMIA LATIFOLIA: Leaves of mountain laurel, *Kalmia latifolia*. Antidiarrheal; also used for skin itches. Principal side effect is vertigo. Contains the poisonous principle grayantoxoin I (for which see RHODODENDRON). [23; also see ref. 21, pp. 100-101]

KASSADER: Same as MECHOACANNA.

KERMES: Pregnant female of insect *Coccus ilicis* (but once thought to be a berry), collected from an evergreen oak,

Quercus coccifera, and used to make the scarlet dye that Pope Paul II prescribed in 1464 to replace the traditional Tyrian purple for coloring cardinals' robes. Mild astringent and tonic (especially for the heart); also used to hasten birth and prevent spontaneous abortion. [15]

KERMES MINERALE: A preparation of VITRIOL ANTIMONIUM invented by Dr. Johann Rudolf Glauber of Amsterdam in 1651.

KEYSERI, PILULE: Keyser's pill, made with ACETIS HYDRARGYRUS. [15,23]

KINO, GUM: Red extract from *Pterocarpus marsupium*. Introduced from India and Ceylon to England by Dr. John Fothergill in 1757. Powerful astringent for internal and external use. [23,29]. For other botanical and geographic sources, see JAMAICA EXTRACT and SANGUIS DRACONIS.

KNEE HOLLY: See RUSCUS.

KRAMERIA: Root of rhatany, *Krameria triandra* (or *K. argentea*); discovered in Peru in 1779, and introduced to Spain in 1796, England in 1808, and U.S. about 1816. Gentle tonic and powerful astringent, especially for controlling diarrhea. [29]

KUSSANDER: Same as MECHOACANNA.

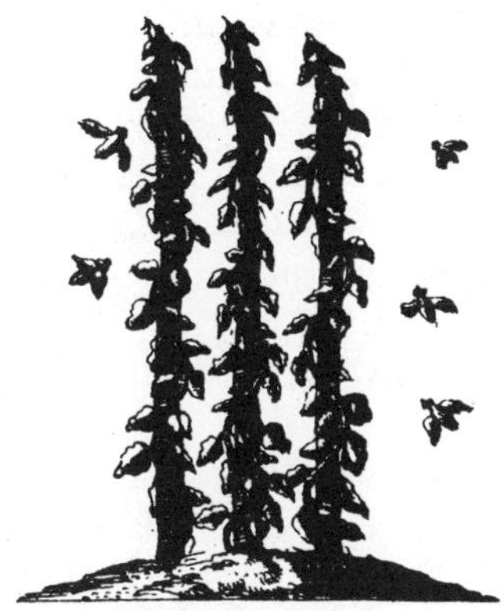

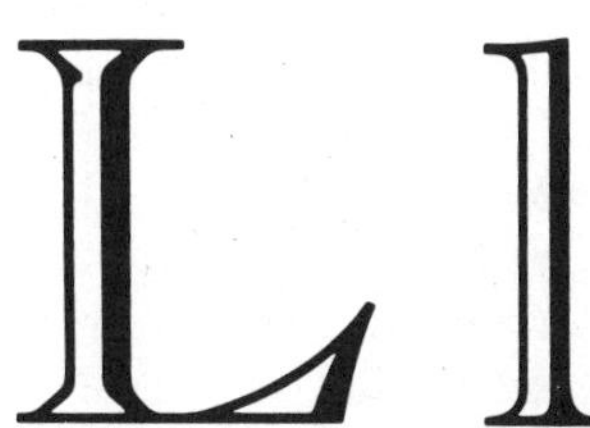

Lacca

LABIALE, CERATUM: "Lip wax," made with OL OLIVA, SPERMACETI, oil of LIGNUM RHODIUM, and CERA ALBA; ALKANET was sometimes added for red color. For chapped lips. [15]

Lac: A milky-appearing drug solution (i.e., an emulsion). [15]

LAC: Milk. Its "inspissated residuum," whey, promotes all natural secretions, and is antiscorbutic, while the whole milk of goats fed on cathartic plants is cathartic.

LACCA (or, sometimes, LAC): Dark red gum resin secreted by female lac insects, *Laccifer lacca*, that live on several southeast Asian tree species (e.g., *Butea frondosa*); when formed into flat thin cakes, it was called "shell-lac." Astringent, especially for scorbutic gums. [15]

LACCAE, TINCTURA: Alcohol extract of LACCA, MYRRH, and COCHLEARIA HORTENSIS. Astringent for bleeding gums; internally, an antiscorbutic, and a corroborant for leukorrhea and gonorrhea (i.e., spermatorrhea). [15]

LAC SULPHURIS: Nearly same as "Flowers of sulphur;" see SULPHUR.

Lactagogue: A drug that stimulates the flow of milk.

LACTUCA: Leaves and seeds of garden lettuce, *Lactuca sativa*, in England, or wild lettuce, *L. virosa*, in Edinburgh (or, sometimes, *L. elongata*). Introduced to medical practice by Dr. Henry Joseph Collin of Vienna in 1771, as a remedy for dropsy. Cooling sedative narcotic that increases the pulse and shares the analgesic, antidiarrheal, and antitussive effects of OPIUM. *L. virosa* was also used as a diuretic, diaphoretic, cathartic, and lactagogue. [2,15,23,29]

LACTUCARIUM: Inspissated juice of LACTUCA. Introduced to medical practice by Dr. John Redman Coxe of Philadelphia in 1799. Soporific, anodyne, and antitussive, like OPIUM, but without its side effects. [29,30]

LAC VIRGINAL: 1) Same as CERUSSA ACETATA. 2) A water suspension of BENZOIN.

LADANI COMPOSITUM, EMPLASTRUM: A stomachic plaster made with LADANUM, FRANKINCENSE, CINNAMOMUM, OL MACIS, and OL MENTHAE. [15]

LADANUM: Aromatic gum resin of *Cistus ladanifer* and perhaps *C. creticus*. Stomachic. [15]

LADIES' MANTLE: See ALCHEMILLA.

LADIES' SMOCK: See CARDAMINE.

Lambative (or Lambitive): A linctus.

LAMBKILL: See KALMIA ANGUSTIFOLIA.

LAPIS CALAMINARIS: Same as CALAMINE.

LAPIS CONTRAYERVAE: "Contrayerva stone," same as PULVIS CONTRAYERVAE COMPOSITUS.

LAPIS GRANCORUM: "Crab stone," same as CANCRORUM LAPILLI.

LAPIS HYBERNICUS: "Irish stone," a black clayey earth containing salts of SULPHUR and FERRUM.

LAPIS INFERNALIS: "Stone of hell," same as ARGENTUM NITRATUM.

LAPIS MEDICAMENTOSUS: "Medical stone." 1) A mixture of astringents based on FERRUM VITRIOLATUM. 2) Same as SAL MURIATICUS.

LAPIS MIRABILIS: "Wonderful stone," a mixture of astringent and vulnerary materials based on VITRIOL.

LARD: Same as AXUNGUENTUM PORCINUM.

LARIX: See PINUS LARIX and OL TEREBINTHA.

LAUDANUM: Usually one of the OPIUM tinctures listed below, but earlier versions included several other non-opiate (and costly) ingredients. The derivation of the word, which was probably invented by Paracelsus, is not certain, although it probably does come from the Latin *laudare*, to praise. The 1820 U.S.P. formula for laudanum contained about 6% OPIUM. Modern laudanum (Opium Tincture, U.S.P., or Deoorized Tincture of Opium) contains 10% opium, or 1.0% morphine.

LAUDANUM LIQUIDUM: Same as TINCTURA THEBAICA.

LAUDANUM LIQUIDUM CYDONIATUM: An alcoholic solution containing 2.8 to 9.4% OPIUM and CINNAMOMUM, NUTMEG, MACE, ACIDUM TARTARI (?), and JUNIPERUS berries; 20 drops produced the same effect as 1 gr. SOLID PANACEA. [3] Cydoniatum means, literally, "with quince," which must have been in the first formula for this tincture.

LAUDANUM, LONDON: A tincture containing about 58% OPIUM, or 1.9-11.3 mg. morphine per recommended dose, depending on body weight, as well as CROCUS, CASTOREUM, OL SUCCINI, MOSCHUS, AMBRAGRISEA, and oil of NUTMEG. [3]

LAUDANUM, SYDENHAM'S: A tincture devised in the 17th century by Dr. Thomas Sydenham of London, it contained 11% OPIUM, as well as CROCUS, CINNAMOMUM, and CARYOPHYLLUS; 20 drops produced the same effect as 1 gr. SOLID PANACEA. [3]

LAUDANUM, WEDEL'S: A strong OPIUM pill formulated much like the SOLID PANACEA, and containing 3.1-12.4 mg. morphine per recommended dose, depending on body weight. Devised in the 17th century by Dr. Georg Wolfgang Wedel of Jena. [3]

LAUREL, MOUNTAIN: See KALMIA LATIFOLIA.

LAUREL, SPURGE: See MEZEREUM.

LAURINUM, UNGUENTUM: "Laurel ointment," made with OVIS and oils of LAURUS, TEREBINTHA, and SUCCINUM. A warm, stimulating ointment, derived from the older formula for UNGUENTUM NERVINUM. [15]

LAURUS: 1) In Europe, bayberries, *Laurus nobilis*. Warm carminative with narcotic and antihysteric properties; used in enemas and fomentations. [15,29] 2) In the U.S., root bark of bayberry, *Myrica pennsylvanica*, or wax myrtle, *M. cerifera*. Used as a mild emetic and as a biliary deobstruent. [23]

LAURUS CAMPHORA: Same as CAMPHOR.

LAURUS CASSIA: Same as CASSIA LIGNEA.

LAURUS CINNAMOMUM: Same as CINNAMOMUM.

LAURUS SASSAFRAS: Same as SASSAFRAS.

LAVANDULA: Same as LAVENDULA.

Lavement: Enema (French).

LAVENDER: See LAVENDULA and STATICE LIMONIUM.

LAVENDER, COMPOUND SPIRITS OF: Solution of LAVENDULA, ROSEMARINUS, CINNAMOMUM, CARYOPHYLLUS, NUTMEG, and HAEMATOXYLUM. Tonic and antirheumatic. [2,15]

LAVENDER, FRENCH: See STECHAS.

LAVENDULA [SPICA]: Flowering spikes of lavender, *Lavandula* spp. Warm tonic and aromatic; also for lice. [15,23,29]

Laxative: A gentle cathartic.

LAXATIVE POWDER: Usually same as MAGNESIA ALBA.

LEAD, SUGAR OF: Same as CERUSSA ACETATA.

LECTISTERNIUM, UNGUENT: An all-purpose unguent for the sickroom. [2] A lectisternium is, literally, "a feast offered to the gods."

LEECHES: see BLEEDING.

LEEK: See PORRUM.

LEE'S NEW LONDON PILLS: Same as LEE'S PILLS, def. no. 2.

LEE'S PILLS: 1) In 1796 Samuel Lee, Jr., of Windham, Conn., was awarded the first American patent for a medicine for his cholagogue "bilious pills," made with ALOES, GAMBOGE, NITER, HERACLEUM, and soap. [7,29] Called Lee's Windham Pills, or Lee's Bilious Pills, they were promoted for jaundice, dysentery, worms, and female complaints, among other indications. 2) Another Lee's Bilious Pill was patented by Samuel H. P. Lee of Plainfield, Conn. In 1830 it contained CALOMEL, JALAP, GAMBOGE, and ANTIMONIUM TARTARISATUM; a later version included ALOES, SCAMMONIUM, GAMBOGE, JALAP, RHAMNUS CATHARTICUS, CALOMEL, and soap. It, too, was a panacea.

LEMERY'S TINCTURE: Made of FERRI RUBIGO and SAL TARTARI (or ACIDUM TARTARICUM). Devised by French pharmaceutical encyclopedist Nicolas Lémery in the mid-18th century. Deobstruent.

LEMNIAN EARTH: A pale red BOLUS that effervesces

slightly with acids. Associated with the Aegean island of Lemnos.

LEMON: See LIMON.

LEMONS, ACID OF: Same as ACIDUM CITRICUM, q.v.

LEMORT'S EXTRACT: Same as TINCTURA OPII CAMPHORATA, with added GLYCERRHIZA, ALKALINE SALT, and honey. LeMort was professor of chemistry at Leyden around 1700. A strong OPIUM preparation containing 3.3-13.0 mg. morphine per recommended dose, depending on body weight. [3,15]

LENIENS, LINCTUS: "Relieving sucker," made with GUM ARABIC, OL AMYGDALA, and AQUA CERASI. For lubricating sore throats. [15]

Lenitive: A soothing or softening medicine, usually a mild cathartic lozenge.

LENTISCUS: Wood of the mastic tree, *Pistachia lentiscus*. Mild astringent, stomachic, tonic, and diuretic. [15] Also see MASTICHE.

LEONARUS CARDIACA: Leaves of motherwort, *Leonurus cardiaca*. Stomachic; antihysteric substitute for OPIUM. [23]

LEONTODON [TARAXACUM]: Same as TARAXACUM.

LEOPARD'S BANE: See ARNICA MONTANA.

LETTUCE: See LACTUCA.

LETTUCE OPIUM: Same as LACTUCARIUM.

Lexipyretus: A febrifuge cataplasm applied to the wrists.

LEY: Same as LYE, but also see CAUSTIC LEY.

LICHEN [ISLANDICUS]: Mucilaginous substance derived from the leaves of Iceland moss, edible liverwort, or eryngo-leaved liverwort, *Lichen islandicus*. Entered medical practice in 1757 on the recommendation of Swedish botanist Dr. Carl von Linné of Uppsala. Nourishing; tonic, astringent, antiseptic, cathartic, and demulcent. [15,30]

LICHEN CINEREUS TERRESTRIS: Leaves of *Peltidea canina*. Diuretic; promoted for treatment of rabies. [15]

LICORICE: See GLYCERRHIZA.

LIGNORUM, DECOCTUM: "Decoction of woods." Same as DECOCTUM GUAIACI COMPOSITUM.

LIGNUM CAMPECHENSE: "Campeche wood," same as HAEMATOXYLUM.

LIGNUM NEPHRITICUM: See NEPHRITICUM LIGNUM.

LIGNUM RHODIUM: "Rosewood," from various spp. of genus *Dalbergia*, perhaps *D. canariensis*. Used chiefly in perfumes, but occasionally in cordials. [15]

LIGNUM VITAE: See GUIAC.

LIGUSTICUM: Seeds of lovage, *Levisticum officinale*. Aromatic. [15]

LILIUM ALBUM: Root of white lily, perhaps *Lilium candidum*. Emollient; sometimes used in poultices. [15]

LILIUM CONVALLIUM: See CONVALLIUM.

LILIUM MINERALE: "Mineral protector," a mixture of sulfides of FERRUM, STANNUM, CUPRUM, and ANTIMONIUM.

LILY OF THE VALLEY: See CONVALLIUM.

LIME: Same as QUICKLIME.

LIME, MURIATE OF: Same as MURIATIS CALCIS.

LIME TREE: See TILIA.

LIME WATER: Same as AQUA CALCIS.

LIMON: Juice or rind of lemon, *Citrus limonia*. Aromatic stomachic; cooling antiseptic; antiemetic; an antidote to OPIUM; not widely recognized as antiscorbutic until the 1790s. Although English naval surgeon Dr. John Woodall had noted its prophylactic value against scurvy as early as 1617, he and Dr. James Lind continued to rely even more heavily on other acids, e.g., VITRIOL, for that purpose. [9,15,23,29,30; John Woodall, *The Surgion's Mate* (1617), p. 185; and Kenneth J. Carpenter, *The History of Scurvy and Vitamin C*, corr. ed. (Cambridge University Press, 1987)] Swedish chemist Karl Wilhelm Scheele isolated citric acid in 1784, but erroneously assumed that it was the antiscorbutic principle of citrus fruits. Ascorbic acid was isolated by Hungarian chemist Albert Szent-Györgyi in 1928-32; it was synthesized in 1933.

LIMONATA SMARAGDINA: "Emerald lemonade," a cordial confection made of emeralds mixed with syrup and seeds of LIMON.

LINARIA: Leaves of toad-flax, spp. of *Linaria*. Weak diuretic and cathartic. [15]

Linctus: A medicine to be licked with the tongue.

LINDEN: See TILIA.

LINGUA CERVINA: Same as SCOLOPENDRIUM.

Liniment: Like an unguent, but further diluted with oil.

LINIMENT DE MINO NEGRO: "Liniment of black lead," made of RED LEAD, OXYMEL OF SQUILLS, and CERATE. [2]

LINIMENT, SAPO: "Soap liniment," mixture of SAPO, CAMPHOR, OL ROSEMARINUS, and ALCOHOL. [2]

LINIMENT, SIMPLE: Made with 4 parts OL OLIVA and 1 part CERA ALBA; cf. SIMPLE OINTMENT. [2]

LINI, OL: Linseed oil; see LINUM. Its principal fatty acid, linoleic acid, was isolated in 1865.

LINUM [USITATISSIMUM]: Seeds, and their oil, of common flax, *Linum usitatissimum*. Used as a demulcent in catarrh, and as a topical emollient for enemas and CANTHARIS-induced blisters; the ground seeds were also used in making poultices. [1,15,30]

LINUM CATHARTICUM: Leaves of purging flax, *Linum catharticum*. Mild cathartic. [15]

Lipara: Unguents or liniments.

LIQUEUR DE PELLEGRIN: A caustic made with ANTIMONIUM MURIATUM and SULPHUR.

LIQUEUR FUMANTE: "Fuming liquid," made of ANTIMONIUM, STANNUM, and HYDRARGYRUS MURIATUS CORROSIVUS.

LIQUIDAMBRA: Resin from trees of *Liquidambar* spp. Aromatic; occasionally used as a substitute for STYRAX, q.v. [15]

LIQUID PANACEA: see PANACEA, LIQUID.

LIQUORITIA: Licorice; see GLYCERRHIZA.

LIRIODENDRON TULIPIFERA: Root bark of tulip tree, or tulip poplar, *Liriodendron tulipifera*. Bitter tonic, antiseptic, and diaphoretic. [23,29,30]

LISBON DIET DRINK: Same as DECOCTUM SARSAPARILLAE COMPOSITUM; introduced as an antivenereal.

LITHARGE: Same as WHITE LEAD.

LITHARGYRI ACETATI, AQUA: Aqueous solution of CERUSSA ACETATA for external use only. [15]

LITHARGYRI CUM HYDRARGYRI, EMPLASTRUM: "Plaster of white lead with mercury." Nearly same as EMPLASTRUM HYDRARGYRI.

LITHARGYRUS: Same as PLUMBUM.

Lithontriptic: A drug that dissolves lithic acid (i.e., uric acid) stones in the urinary tract.

Litus: A liniment.

LIVERWORT: See HEPATICA and LICHEN.

LIXIVA, LIXIVE, LIXIVIA, or LIXIVIUM: When used alone, denotes potash, or potassium carbonate, prepared by burning plant material with close smothering heat; however, after about 1790 the term was also sometimes applied to LYE, potassium hydroxide (sometimes still called caustic potash). Deobstruent, attenuant, diaphoretic, antacid, diuretic, and aperient. [1,2,15,23]

LIXIVA ACETATA: Potassium acetate. Mild cathartic; strong diuretic. [15]

LIXIVA NITRATA: Same as SAL NITRITI.

LIXIVA SULPHUREA: Same as KALI SULPHURATUM.

LIXIVA TARTARI[SATA]: Same as SAL TARTARI.

LIXIVA VITRIOLATA: Same as KALI SULPHURATUM.

LOBELIA [INFLATA]: Leaves of Indian tobacco, or emetic weed, *Lobelia inflata*. Emetic; sometimes cathartic; diaphoretic and expectorant in small doses. Because it can cause death during convulsions, it is considered too hazardous for routine clinical use. Its effects are like those of tobacco (see NICOTIANA). [23,29,30] Lobelia was the keystone of the system of botanic medicine promoted by Samuel Thomson from about 1806. [15,23; see Thomson's *New Guide to Health, or Botanic Family Physician*, 1822, and many subsequent editions; J. Worth Estes and David M. Goodman, *The Changing Humors of Portsmouth* (Boston: Countway Library of Medicine, 1986), pp. 59-69] In 1813, Rev. Manasseh Cutler of Massachusetts promoted the drug's value in asthma; it entered British medical practice in 1829. Lobeline, which has properties like those of nicotine but is less potent, was isolated from *L. inflata* by Procter in 1838-41, and crystallized by German chemist Heinrich Wieland in 1915. Although used as a respiratory stimulant in the early 20th century, lobeline has no therapeutic value.

LOBELIA SYPHILITICA: Leaves of great blue lobelia, *Lobelia syphilitica*. Emetic, cathartic, and diuretic; ineffective in syphilis. [23]

LOCATELLI, LOCATELLUS, or LUCATELLI, BALSAM OF: Expensive preparation containing CERA FLAVA, OL OLIVA, TEREBINTHA, and SANGUIS DRACONIS or SANTALUM RUBRUM. Emollient and astringent. [2]

LOCKYER'S PILLS: A proprietary remedy invented by a "licensed physitian" of London about 1660, it was a mixture of PANACEA ANTIMONII, GUM TRAGACANTH, and sugar. Cathartic and emetic. [14,15]

LOGWOOD: Same as HAEMATOXYLUM.

Lohoch: Virtually the same as a looch, linctus, or electuary.

LONDON LAUDANUM: See LAUDANUM, LONDON.

Looch: A thick pectoral remedy sucked from the end of a licorice (GLYCERRHIZA) stick.

LOOSESTRIFE: See LYTHRUM SALICARIA.

LOPEZ TREE: See INDICA LOPEZIANA.

LORDS-AND-LADIES: See COSMETIC UNGUENT.

LOVAGE: See LIGUSTICUM.

Lozenge: A troche.

LUCE, EAU DE (or AQUA LUCCANA, AQUA LUCII, AQUA SANCTI LUCIAE, etc.): Same as SPIRITUS AMMONIAE SUCCINATUS; named for the 18th-century pharmacist who invented it in Lille, France, although the name was later corrupted (e.g., to "St. Lucy's water.") An inhalant for fainting and hysteria.

LUCIS MAJORIS, PILULE: "Pill for better eyesight," a collyrium made with 37 ingredients.

LUGOL'S SOLUTION: Aqueous solution of IODINE and potassium iodide invented in the early 19th century by French physician Jean G.–A. Lugol. Antiseptic. Now used chiefly in tissue staining.

LUJULA: Leaves of wood sorrel, *Oxalis acetosella*. Properties like those of ACETOSA, but more agreeable. Refrigerant; thirst-quencher. [15] Contains SAL ACETOSELLAE.

LUNAR CAUSTIC: "Silver caustic," ARGENTUM NITRATUM.

LUNARE, PILULE: "Silver pill," made with recrystallized silver nitrate. Caustic, but milder than ARGENTUM NITRATUM; mild cathartic; anthelminthic. [15]

LUPINUS: Seeds of white lupine, *Lupinus albus*. Anthelminthic, but can produce severe side effects. [15]

LUPULUS: Flower of the common hop, *Humulus lupulus*. A strong bitter astringent with tonic, narcotic, soporific, and anodyne properties; used in malt liquors as a stomachic; antaphrodisiac. [15,23,29,30]

LYCOPERDON: Puff ball mushrooms, *Lycoperdon* spp. Applied to wounds to stop bleeding. [15]

LYCOPUS: Bugleweed, *Lycopus virginicus*, or water-horehound, *L. americanus*. Mild astringent, narcotic, and antitussive; sedates the circulation. [29]

LYE: 1) Potassium hydroxide; see LIXIVA. 2) Sodium hydroxide. Lithontriptic; antacid. [15]

LYE, CAUSTIC: Potassium hydroxide; see AQUA POTASSAE.

LYTHRUM SALICARIA: Purple, or spiked, loosestrife, *Lythrum salicaria*. Demulcent and astringent antidiarrheal. [29]

LYTTA VITTATA: See CANTHARIS.

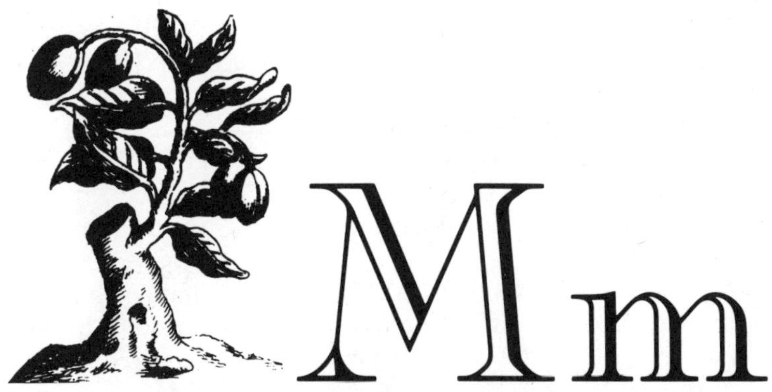

Moschata

M: Abbreviation for *Misce*, "mix," used in prescription writing.

MACE or MACIS: see NUTMEG.

MACRI, PILULE: Stimulates the stomach, brain, nerves, and muscles.

MADDER: See RUBIA.

MAGGOTS: Fly larvae. Occasionally used, since the 16th century at least, to clean gangrenous wounds. [Eli Chernin, "Surgical maggots," *Southern Medical Journal 79* (1986): 1143-1145]

Magistery: 1) A substance precipitated from an acid solution. 2) An especially prepared medicine.

MAGISTERY OF BISMUTH: Same as SUBNITRAS BISMUTHI.

MAGISTERY OF JOVE (or JUPITER): Acetate of STANNUM.

MAGISTERY OF SATURN: Same as WHITE LEAD.

MAGISTERY OF TARTAR: Same as POTASSAE, ACETIS.

Magma: A soft ointment or confection.

MAGNANIMITATIS, AQUA: "Water of magnanimity." Made with FORMICAE CUM ACERVO.

MAGNES ARSENICALIS: "Arsenical magnet," a gentle caustic for syphilitic chancres made of WHITE ARSENIC, SULPHUR, and ANTIMONIUM.

MAGNESIA: Same as MAGNESIA USTA.

MAGNESIA ALBA: Magnesium carbonate. Strong antacid cathartic and antilithic. [1,2,15,23,29,30]

MAGNESIAE CARBONAS: Same as MAGNESIA ALBA.

MAGNESIAE SULPHAS: Same as MAGNESIA VITRIOLATA.

MAGNESIA NIGRA: Manganese.

MAGNESIA OPALINA: A form of ANTIMONIUM prepared with SAL MURIATICUS and NITER.

MAGNESIA USTA: Magnesium oxide. Gastric antacid. [1,2,15,23].

MAGNESIA VITRIOLATA: Magnesium sulfate. A mild cathartic, diuretic, and diaphoretic. Isolated in 1695 by Dr. Nehemiah Grew from the medicinal water discovered in 1616 at Epsom Wells in Surrey, England. [1,2,15,23]

MAGNETICUM, EMPLASTRUM: A penetrating and suppurative plaster made with MAGNES ARSENICALIS.

MAGNOLIA: Extract of *Magnolia glauca* (and perhaps other species). Sedative, diaphoretic, and tonic. [1,29,30]

MAJORANA: Leaves of marjoram, *Majorana hortensis.* Tonic, cephalic, and expectorant; powder used as an errhine. [15,29]

Malactica: Emollient remedies.

Malagmata: Cataplasms or other external antiseptics.

MALE FERN: See FILIX.

MALLOW, MARSH: See ALTHAEA.

MALLOW, MUSK: See MALVA SYLVESTRIS.

MALTHACODE, EMPLASTRUM: "Tar plaster," made with CERA ALBA and TEREBINTHA or PIX.

MALVA [SYLVESTRIS]: Leaf and flower of musk mallow, *Malva moschata.* Mild cathartic; used chiefly in emollient enemas; also used in cataplasms. [15,23,29]

MANDRAGORA (or MANDRAKE): 1) Root of *Atropa mandragora.* Although historically classified as a sedative narcotic, and purported to be an aphrodisiac, it has little discernible effect, even if it does contain a modest amount of scopolamine, an antimuscarinic alkaloid. [15; also see Charles B. Heiser, Jr., *Nightshades: the Paradoxical Plants* (San Francisco: W.H. Freeman, 1967), pp. 129-136] 2) In North America, same as PODOPHYLLUM PELTATUM.

MANNA ASH: Same as GUM MANNA.

MANNA, GUM: Resin of *Fraxinus ornus.* Weak demulcent cathartic and expectorant; produces intestinal gas and colic. [2,15,23,29] Mannose and mannitol, now used as an osmotic diuretic, were first isolated from this plant.

MANNA THURIS: 1) Same as THUS. 2) A coarse form of OLIBANUM.

MANUS CHRISTI: "Hand of Christ;" same as DIAMARGARITUM SIMPLEX.

MANUS DEI: "Hand of God," a plaster made with MYRRH, OLIBANUM, GALBANUM, and GUM AMMONIAC.

MARANTA ARUNDINACEA: Root of West Indian arrowroot, *Maranta arundinacea.* Introduced from Jamaica to England in early 18th century. A nutritious and mucilaginous starch suitable for the sick, especially those with diarrhea. [23,29,30]

MARCHIONIS, PULVIS: "Marchioness' powder;" same as PULVIS AD GUTTETAM.

MARCOST ASHES: Same as LIXIVA.

MARGARITAE: Pearls. Cordial and tonic. However, they had disappeared from most practices by the late 18th century.

MARIGOLD: See CALENDULA.

MARIJUANA: See CANNABIS.

MARINI, SPIRITUS SALIS: "Spirits of sea salt," same as SAL MURIATICUS.

MARINUS HISPANUS, SAL: "Spanish sea salt," same as SAL MURIATICUS.

MARJORAM: See MAJORANA.

MARMOR: Marble, a form of calcium carbonate, which is also the medicinally active component of CRETA (chalk).

MARRUBIUM [VULGARE]: Leaves of white horehound, *Marrubium vulgare.* Aperient, cathartic, attenuant, diuretic, diaphoretic, and, especially, expectorant. [15,23,29]

MARS: Iron; see FERRUM.

MARS, BALLS OF (or BOULES DE MARS): A complex preparation of FERRUM TARTARISATUM.

MARSEILLES VINEGAR: Same as ACETUM AROMATICUM, but see VINAIGRE DES QUATRE VOLEURS for the Marseilles connection.

MARSH MALLOW: See ALTHAEA.

MARSH TREFOIL: See TRIFOLIUM PALUDOSUM.

MARS SOLUBILIS: "Soluble iron." Same as FERRUM TARTARISATUM.

MARS TARTARISATUS: Same as FERRUM TARTARISATUM.

MARTIAL FLOWERS: Same as FERRUM AMMONIATUM.

MARTIALIS, CROCUS: Same as FERRI RUBIGO.

MARTIALIS, SAL: Same as FERRUM AMMONIATUM.

MARTIAL SAFFRON: Same as SUB-CARBONAS FERRI.

MARTIATUM, UNGUENTUM: "Soldier's unguent," a green ointment made with LAURUS, RUTA, MAJORANA, MENTHA, SALVIA and ABSINTHUM VULGARE.

MARTIS, EXTRACTUM: Same as VINUM FERRI, but evaporated further to increase the concentration of iron. [15]

MARUM SYRIACUM: Syrian herb mastic, *Teucrium marum*. Errhine. [15]

MASSICOT: Same as WHITE LEAD.

MASTERWORT: See HERACLEUM and IMPERATORIA.

MASTIC, GUM: Same as MASTICHE.

MASTICHE: Gum mastic, resin of *Pistacia lentiscus* tree. Tonic and astringent. [15] Used only to fill dental cavities by mid-19th century. [29] Also see LENTISCUS.

MASTICHINAE, PILULE: Cathartic pill made with MASTICHE, ABSINTHUM VULGARE, HIERA PICRA, and ALOES.

MASTIC, SYRIAN HERB: See MARUM SYRIACUM.

MATRICARIA: Leaves of common featherfew, or German chamomile, *Tanacetum parthenium*. Antihysteric emmenagogue; bitter tonic, emetic, febrifuge, and antiseptic; anthelminthic in large doses. [15,29]

MATTHEW'S PILL: A proprietary preparation containing 12-14% OPIUM, or 3.0-12.1 mg. morphine per recommended dose, depending on body weight, as well as IRIS FLORENTINA, HELLEBORUS ALBUS, HELLEBORUS NIGER, ACIDUM TARTARICUM, TEREBINTHA, and soap. [3]

MAY APPLE: Same as PODOPHYLLUM PELTATUM.

MAYWEED: See COTULA FOETIDA.

MEADOW SAFFRON: See COLCHICUM.

MEADOWSWEET: See ULMARIA.

Measurement: The 1794 *Edinburgh Dispensatory* lamented that the use of two different systems of weight had caused great confusion in the preparation of medicines. The London and

Edinburgh pharmacopoeias specified that Troy weights (named for Troyes, France, where frequent medieval fairs necessitated the development of a common system of mensuration) be used in compounding and dispensing medicines; thus, Troy (or troy) weights are also called Apothecaries' weights. Sometimes it was called the Goldsmiths' system, because jewellers defined their carat as 3.168 Troy grains (although they also defined 1 carat of gold as 1/24 part of the whole). The units of Troy weight are:

1 pound	= 12 ounces	= 5760 grains	(= 373.242 grams)
1 ounce	= 8 drachms	= 480 grains	(= 31.103 grams)
1 drachm	= 3 scruples	= 60 grains	(= 3.888 grams)
1 scruple	=	20 grains	(= 1.296 grams)
1 grain			(= 0.648 grams)

Although this system had originally been based on the weight of a grain of wheat, the standard pound adopted by the British Parliament in 1760 was retained by the United States even after they became independent.

By contrast, wholesale druggists (and others, e.g., grocers) used the Avoirdupois system:

1 pound	= 16 ounces	= 7000 grains	(= 453.592 grams)
1 ounce	= 16 drachms	= 437.5 grains	(= 28.350 grams)
1 drachm		= 27.344 grains	(= 1.772 grams)
1 grain			(= 64.799 milligrams)

Thus, 18th-century pharmacists bought their raw materials for compounding medicines by the pound Avoirdupois, but manufactured them by Troy (Apothecaries') weight.

When the London College of Physicians adopted Troy weights for medicines in 1618, they also adopted the following system of liquid measures:

1 gallon =	8 pints
1 pint =	16 [fluid]ounces
1 ounce =	8 [flui]drachms
1 drachm =	60 minims, to replace the older, and all too variable, drops [gutta]

However, because the densities of many liquids varied (they were least for the purest alcohols, and greatest for the concentrated acids), the Edinburgh College specified that liquids be weighed rather than measured volumetrically.

In 1826 the British Parliament defined the Imperial gallon as 10 lb. Avoirdupois of distilled water at 62° F. and 30 in. barometric pressure. The minim is still defined in Great Britain as 0.00361 cu. in.; in the U.S., the equivalent volume, 1/60 fluidrachm, is 0.00376 cu. in. In 1836, the U. S. Congress directed the Secretary of the Treasury to furnish every state with standards of both the Troy and Avoirdupois pounds made according to current British specifications. However, the volume of the U.S. gallon (231 cu. in., or 58,372.2 gr. distilled water weighed at 62°F. and 30 in. barometric pressure) is only 80% of the volume of the British, or Imperial, gallon.

Although James Watt had suggested the metric system as early as 1783, it was not adopted by any country until the French National Assembly did in 1793. It was legalized, although not made compulsory, in Britain in 1864, and in the U.S. two years later. Metric measurements were incorporated by the *U.S. Pharmacopoeia* in 1890, and by the *British Pharmacopoeia* in 1914. By an Executive Order of 1893, American customary measures were defined in international metric terms:

1 lb. Avoirdupois = 453.5924277 gm.;
1 lb. Apothecary (or Troy) = 5760/7000 lb. Avoirdupois; and
1 liquid quart Apothecary (or Wine) = 0.946 L.
(1 liquid Imperial quart now = 1.1359 L.)

Compendia such as dispensatories and pharmacopoeias used whichever system was currently in force in the time and place in which they were written, unless otherwise specified. Most pharmacists and physicians followed suit in their prescriptions, daybooks, ledgers, letters, and other documents.

Common symbols and abbreviations used to denote Troy medical measurements include:

Pound [libra]: ℔	(later, #)
Ounce [uncia]: ℥	(later, Oz.)
Drachm [drachma]: ʒ	(later, Dr., Dram)
Scruple [scrupulus]: ℈	
Grain [grana]: Gr.	

Gallon [congius]: Cong. (later, Gal.)
Pint [octarius]: (later, Pt.)
Fluidounce [fluiduncia]: *f* ℥
Fluidrachm [fluidrachma]: *f* ʒ
Half of any of the above: ss.
Minims [minima]: ♍
Drops [gutta]: Gtt.
A spoonful [cochleare]: Coch.

Directions for taking liquid medicines have been given to patients in terms of convenient and familiar household objects for many centuries (e.g., ancient Egyptians prescribed in terms of the *ro*, which was about half an ounce, a modern tablespoonful):

1 glassful	=	8 ounces	=	240 ml.
1 teacupful	=	4 ounces	=	120 ml.
1 wineglassful	=	2 ounces	=	60 ml.
2 tablespoonfuls	=	1 ounce	=	30 ml.
1 tablespoonful	=	1/2 ounce	=	15 ml.
1 teaspoonful	=	1/4 ounce	=	5 ml.

For 18th-century discussions of weights and volumetric measures, see ref. 15, pp. 56-59, and ref. 23, pp. 90-92. For tables of equivalent measures in Great Britain and the U.S., see Samuel W. Goldstein, "Metrology," in Eric W. Martin, ed., *Remington's Pharmaceutical Sciences*, ed. 13 (Easton, Penna.: Mack Publishing Co., 1965), pp. 81-87, and other tables in the same volume. For the early origins of most measurements, see Ronald Edward Zupko, "Medieval Apothecary Weights and Measures: the Principal Units of England and France," *Pharmacy in History 32* (1990): 57-62.]

MECCA, BALM OF: Usually, same as BALM OF GILEAD, but may sometimes be an extract of *Balsamodendron gileadense*, used for similar purposes.

MECHAMECK: Same as MECHOACANNA.

MECHOACANNA: Root of wild potato, or mechoacan, *Ipomoea mechoacanna* (although sometimes, rarely, JALAP). Weak cathartic and diuretic. [15,23,29,30]

MECONIUM, or MECONIO, SYRUP E: "Poppy juice." Same as DIACODIUM.

Mel: A mixture of active drug ingredient(s) with honey.

MEL: Same as HONEY.

MELALEUCA LEUCADENDRON: See CAJEPUT.
MELAMPODIUM: Same as HELLEBORUS NIGER.
Melanagoga: Remedies that purge black bile or melancholy.
MEL DESPUMATUM: Clarified honey.
MELIA AZEDARACH: Fruit and root of chinaberry, *Melia azedarach*. Introduced to Europe by Dr. Garcia d'Orta, Portuguese physician at Goa, in 1563. Anthelminthic. Side effects include mydriasis, coma, difficult breathing, vomiting, and diarrhea, but said not to be fatal (however, see ref. 21, pp. 115-116). [23,29,30]
Melicratium: Same as Hydromel.
MELIMELUM: Conserve of CYDONIA MALUS (or other apple-like fruit) in honey.
MELISSA [OFFICINALIS]: Balm gentle or balm mint, *Melissa officinalis*. Weak tonic, antihysteric, and diluent. [15]
MELISSAE, AQUA: "Mint water." Same as AQUA CARMELITANA.
MELLILOT: Leaves and flowers of sweet clover, *Melilotus alba* and *M. officinalis*. Used in emollient glysters and cataplasms, for abdominal and uterine inflammations. [2,15] When spoiled as silage, sweet clover yields dicumarol, used since the 1940s as an anticoagulant.
MELLI OPTIMI: The best grade of honey. Used especially in sore throat remedies, and sometimes in skin unguents. [1,2]
Mellita: Medicated honeys, such as Mels and Oxymels.
MELOE VESICATORIUS: Same as CANTHARIS.
Menstruum: A solvent (e.g., VINUM) used in extracting drugs.
MENTHA: When used alone, usually means MENTHA PIPERITA.
MENTHA CATARIA: Same as NEPETA.
MENTHA PIPERITA: Leaves of peppermint, *Mentha piperita*. Introduced to medicine in England in late 17th century. Warm tonic, carminative, and antispasmodic. [1,2,15,23,29,30] Also see ESSENCE OF PEPPERMINT.
MENTHA PULEGIUM: Same as PULEGIUM.
MENTHA SATIVA (or VIRIDIS): Leaves of spearmint, *Mentha spicata*. A warm carminative, stomachic, antihysteric, antiemetic, and antilienteric. [15,23]
MENYANTHES: Same as TRIFOLIUM PALUDOSUM.
MERCURIAL INJECTION: A medication made of a salt of HYDRARGYRUS and administered with a PENIS SYRINGE.

MERCURIALIS: Leaves of herb mercury, *Mercurialis annua*. Mild cathartic, usually administered by enema. [15]

MERCURIALIS, AQUA: "Mercury water." Same as MERCURIUS LIQUIDUS.

MERCURIALIS SIMPLEX, SOLUTIO: "Simple solution of mercury," a mixture of HYDRARGYRUS PURIFICATUS, GUM ARABIC (or GUM TRAGACANTH), KERMES, and FUMARIA, sometimes with honey added. Devised (or perhaps simply promoted) by late 18th-century Viennese dermatologist Joseph Jacob von Plenck. For skin disorders. [15]

MERCURIAL OINTMENTS: Unguents for syphilitic chancres, or for itch, made with, e.g., HYDRARGYRUS PURIFICATUS, HYDRARGYRUS NITRATUS RUBER, or WHITE PRECIPITATE. [2,12]

MERCURIAL PILLS: Used for syphilis, or to produce catharsis; see HYDRARGYRUS. Typical formulations included: HYDRARGYRUS PURIFICATUS, CONSERVE OF RED ROSES, and starch or GLYCERRHIZA [2]; HYDRARGYRUS PURIFICATUS and HONEY rubbed together until the globules of mercury disappear, SAPO ALBUS, and GUM AMMONIAC [12]; and HYDRARGYRUS PURIFICATUS and GUM MANNA [15]. The term might also be applied to any mercury-containing pill, e.g., CALOMEL.

MERCURIC PRECIPITATE RUBRUM: Red mercuric oxide. Escharotic. [2]

MERCURIC SUBLIMATE: Same as HYDRARGYRUS MURIATUS CORROSIVUS.

MERCURII CINEREUS, PULVIS: Same as HYDRARGYRUS PRAECIPITATUS.

MERCURIUS: See HYDRARGYRUS.

MERCURIUS ALKALISATUS: "Alkaline mercury," made of HYDRARGYRUS PURIFICATUS and CANCRORUM LAPILLI (a combination like that in HYDRARGYRUS CUM CRETA).

MERCURIUS DULCIS: Same as CALOMEL.

MERCURIUS LIQUIDUS: HYDRARGYRUS dissolved in nitric acid. Applied externally to skin sores. [15]

MERCURIUS PRAECIPITATUS RUBER: Same as HYDRARGYRUS NITRATUS RUBER.

MERCURIUS VITAE: "Mercury of life." Recrystallized

ANTIMONIUM MURIATUM, but actually antimony oxychloride ($SbOCl$).

MERCURY: See HYDRARGYRUS.

Mesenterica: Appetite stimulants used to treat disorders of the mesentery.

METALLICUM, SAL: Same as LILIUM MINERALE.

METALLORUM, CROCUS: Same as CROCUS ANTIMONII, but the original 17th–century formula included SAL NITER and wine.

Metrenchytum: A syringe for injecting drugs into the uterus.

MEUM: Root of spignel, or baldmoney, *Meum athamanticum*. Aromatic stimulant and carminative. [15]

MEZEREUM (or MEZEREON) : Bark of root of spurge laurel, or mezereon, *Daphne mezereon*. Tonic and diuretic. Side effects include burning in the mouth, vomiting, and catharsis. Also used as a blister for tumors and non-venereal cutaneous eruptions. [15,23,29]

MICA PANIO: Bread crumbs, taken internally in water for treating many gastrointestinal symptoms, or applied externally as a plaster to stimulate suppuration. [1]

MICA THURIS: "Crumbs of frankincense." A finely powdered form of OLIBANUM.

Micleta: An astringent remedy for bleeding and hemorrhoids.

Migma: A mixture of several drugs.

MILK: Same as LAC.

MILLE FLORUM: "Thousand flowers," same as AQUA FLORUM OMNIUM.

MILLEFOLIUM: Leaves and flowers of yarrow, *Achillea millefolium*. Mild astringent for internal and external use; antihysteric, tonic, and sedative. [15]

MILLEPEDA: Dried and powdered woodlice, crawling arthropods of class Diplopoda, with double pairs of legs attached to most body segments. Diuretic and deobstruent; the conserve was sometimes recommended especially for children. [15]

MIMOSA CATECHU: Same as CATECHU.

MIMOSA NILOTICA: See GUM ARABIC and ACACIA VERA.

MINDERERUS, SPIRITS [or TINCTURE] OF: Nearly same as AQUA AMMONIAE ACETATAE. Introduced by Dr. Raymond Minderer of Augsburg in 1610 as a cathartic and diaphoretic. [2,13,15]

Minims (or Minima): Units of volume; see Measurement.

MINIUM: Same as RED LEAD.

MINT: See MENTHA entries, and PULEGIUM.

MINT, BALM: See MELISSA OFFICINARUM.

MINT, HORSE: See MONARDA.

MIRABILE GLAUBERI, SAL: "Glauber's" wonderful salt. Same as GLAUBER'S SALT.

MIRANDOLAE, PULVIS PRINCIPIS: "Powder of the Prince of Mirandola," i.e., Giovanni Pico, the 15th-century count of Mirandola whose writings presaged some of Paracelsus's ideas. Nearly same as GOUT POWDER OF DUKE OF PORTLAND.

MISTLETOE: See VISCUS.

MITHRIDATE, or MITHRADATUM: A relatively weak OPIUM preparation said to have been invented in the 2nd century B.C. by Mithradates VI, king of Pontus. It was usually made from about 50 ingredients, but often many more. A formula used in 1701 contained 0.3% OPIUM, or 2.3-9.4 mg. morphine per recommended dose, depending on body weight. [3,13] Although Dr. William Heberden of London had noted in 1795 that mithridate's formula called only for RUTA, SAL MURIATICUS, CARICA, and two nuts, a 1794 Edinburgh formula included: cinnamon, myrrh, agaric, Indian nard, ginger, saffron, seeds of mithridate mustard, frankincense, Chio turpentine, camel's hay, costus (or zedoary), Indian leaf (or mace), stechas, long pepper, hartwort seeds, hypocistis, storax, opoponax, galbanum, opobalsam (or oil of nutmeg), castor, poley mountain, scordium, carpobalsam (or cubebs), white pepper, candy carrot seed, bdellium, Celtic nard, gentian, dittany of Crete, red roses, Macedonian parsley seed, lesser cardamon seeds, sweet fennel seeds, gum arabic, opium, calamus aromaticus, valerian, anise seed, sagapenum, meum athamanticum, St. John's wort, acacia (or terra japonica), bellies of skinks, and clarified honey. These 45 ingredients—not all of which are defined in this dictionary—were difficult to formulate into a powder. [15, pp. 550-551; also see Gilbert Watson, *Theriac and Mithradatium* (London: Wellcome Historical Medical Library, 1966)]

Mochlica: Drugs that purge violently both ways (i.e., as vomiting and catharsis).

MONARDA: Horsemint, *Monarda punctata*. Stimulant carminative, diaphoretic, and antiemetic. [29,30] Contains thymol (see THYMUS).

Monohemera: Remedies that heal in only one day.

MORPHINE: See OPIUM.

MORRAIN, UNGUENT: An unguent for horses and other animals with a murrain, any of several epidemic diseases of farm animals.

MORUS (or MORA): Fruit of the mulberry, *Morus* spp. (perhaps *M. rubra*). Cooling, aperient, diuretic, and diaphoretic; the bark is anthelminthic. [15,29]

MOSCHATA: See NUX MOSCHATA MARE.

MOSCHATA, MISTURA: Made with NUTMEG, GUM ARABIC, sugar, and ROSE water. [15]

MOSCHUS [MOSCHIFERUS]: Musk, the odorous secretion produced by a gland beneath the abdominal skin of the male Asian musk deer, *Moscus moschiferus*, and now used in perfumery. Stimulant anticonvulsive, antispasmodic, diaphoretic, analgesic, sedative, and antihysteric; increases the pulse "without heating much." Given to children as an enema. [15,23,29,30]

MOTHER-OF-PEARL: Powdered iridescent lining of several mollusk shells. Cephalic, cordial, analeptic, pectoral, and styptic.

MOTHER-OF-THYME: See SERPYLLUM.

MOTHER'S OINTMENT: Made by pouring powdered WHITE LEAD into melted OVIS, AXUNGUENTUM PORCINUM, and butter.

MOTHERWORT: See LEONARUS CARDIACA.

MOULT'S BITTER PURGING SALTS: A proprietary preparation of MAGNESIA VITRIOLATA.

MUCILAGINOUS MIXTURE: Powdered GUM ARABIC administered in warm water, CONSERVE OF ROSES, or ALTHAEA, to relieve sore throat. [1]

Mucilago: A glutinous substance, usually a concentrated aqueous solution of starch or certain gums.

MUCUNA: Same as DOLICHOS.

MUGWORT: See ARTEMISIA.

MULBERRY: See MORUS.

MULLEIN: See VERBASCUM.

Mulsa, Aqua: Same as Hydromel.

MUMMY: Powdered Egyptian mummy, used (symbolically or sympathetically) as a restorative tonic. [ref. 8, p. 113; also see Thomas Joseph Pettigrew, *A History of Egyptian Mummies* (London: 1834), pp. 1-12]

MUNDIFICATIVUM, UNGUENTUM: "Cleansing ointment."

MURIA: Same as SAL MURIATICUS.

MURIAS: A salt of ACIDUM MURIATICUM.

MURIAS AMMONIAE: Same as SAL AMMONIAC.

MURIAS AMMONIAE ET FERRI: A crude form of FERRUM AMMONIATUM.

MURIAS ANTIMONII: Same as ANTIMONIATUM MURIATUM.

MURIAS BARYTAE: Barium chloride. Tonic, diaphoretic, and diuretic in small doses; large doses produce vertigo, emesis, catharsis, tremors, and coma. Also used externally as a gentle escharotic for cutaneous conditions. [23,30]

MURIAS CALCIS: Calcium chloride. Tonic. Side effects include nausea and vomiting. [23]

MURIAS HYDRARGYRI: Same as CALOMEL.

MURIAS SODAE: Same as SAL MURIATICUS.

MURIATICUM, ACIDUM: Hydrochloric acid. When appropriately diluted, it is antiphlogistic, tonic, refrigerant, antiseptic, aperient, and diuretic. [23,29]

MURIATICUS, SAL: Sea salt, sodium chloride. Warm and dry tonic, antiseptic, appetite stimulant, digestive, styptic, cathartic, emetic, and anthelminthic, depending on dose. Often used in enemas. [15]

MUSA AENEA: Literally, "copper muse." A soporific made with OPIUM.

MUSK: See ABELMOSCHUS and MOSCHUS.

MUSTARD: See SINAPI.

MUTTON SUET: See OVIS.

MYNSICHT'S APERITIVE MARTIAL MAGISTERY: Made with filtrate of boiled TAMARINDUS and FERRI LIMATURA PURIFICATA. Described by German alchemist Adrian Mynsicht of Mecklenburg in 1631. A tonic deobstruent.

MYNSICHT'S BLISTERING PLASTER: Made with CANTHARIS, ZINGIBER, and PIPER LONGUM. Described by Adrian Mynsicht of Mecklenberg in 1631.

MYNSICHT'S CICERA TARTARI: "Peas of tartar," described by Adrian Mynsicht in 1631, was made with ACIDUM TARTARICUM, TEREBINTHA, AQUA

VIOLARUM, NITER, and IRIS FLORENTINA. Deobstruent.

MYNSICHT'S ELIXIR [OF VITRIOL]: Same as ACIDUM VITRIOLI AROMATICUM, but Adrian Mynsicht's 1631 formula included many other aromatics.

MYREPSUS: See REQUIES NICOLAI.

MYRICA CERIFERA [HUMILIS]: See LAURUS, def. 2.

MYRICALIS, PULVIS: An appetite stimulant made with tamarisk (*Tamarix* spp.), which was called *myrica* in Latin.

MYRISTICA [MOSCHATA]: Same as NUTMEG.

MYROBALANI: Dried fruit of myrobolans, *Prunus cerasifera*. Astringent, cathartic. [15]

MYROXYLON [BALSAMUM]: Same as SYRUP OF TOLU.

MYROXYLON PEREIRAE: Same as BALSAM OF PERU.

MYROXYLON PERUIFERA: Same as BALSAM OF PERU.

MYRRH: Gum resin extracted from *Commiphora abyssinica*. Stimulating tonic, diaphoretic, expectorant, stomachic, antidiarrheal, emmenagogue, and antiseptic (especially when applied topically as a tincture). [1,2,23,29,30]

MYRRHAE COMPOSITUM, ELIXIR: Same as TINCTURA SABINAE COMPOSITA.

MYRRHAE COMPOSITUS, PULVIS: "Compound powder of myrrh," made of MYRRH, SAVIN, RUTA, and CASTOR. Emmenagogue. [15]

MYRRHA, TROCHISCI E: A somewhat more complex formulation of PULVIS MYRRHAE COMPOSITUS; originally ascribed to the late 9th-century physician Rhazes. [15]

MYRTLE: See MYRTUS.

MYRTLE, WAX: See LAURUS, def. no. 2.

MYRTUS: Berries of myrtle, *Myrtus communis*. Internally, astringent, antiseptic, and sedative; externally, stimulant and antiseptic. [15]

MYRTUS PIMENTA: Same as PIMENTO.

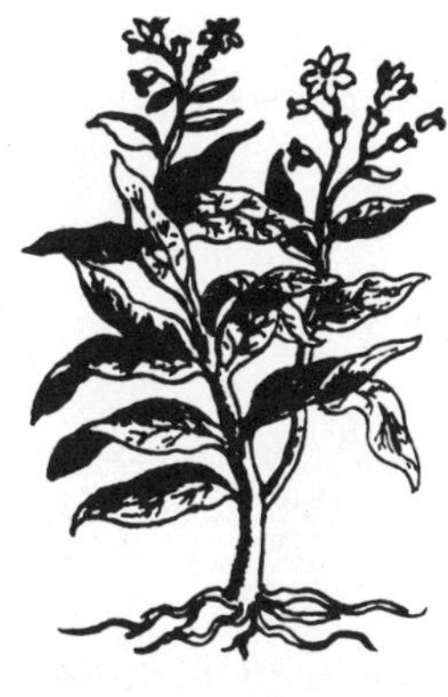
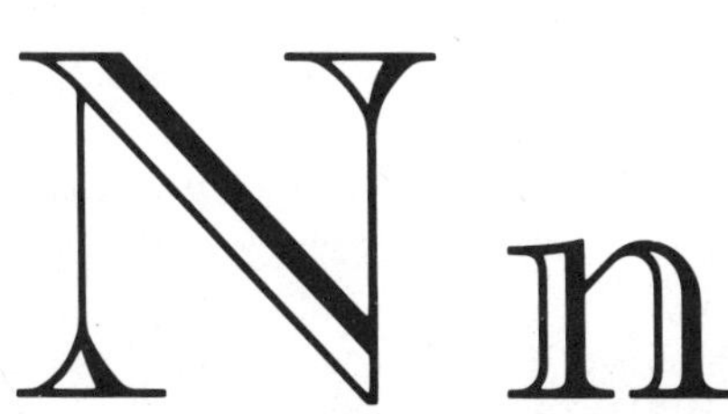

Nicotiana

NANCY, BOULES DE: "Balls of Nancy," same as BALLS OF MARS.

NAPELLUM: Same as ACONITUM.

NAPHAE, AQUA: Distilled water of flowers of AURANTIUM.

NAPHTHA: Same as PETROLEUM.

NAPUS: Seeds of navew, or rape, *Brassica napus*. Attenuating, detergent, and alexipharmic. [15]

Narcotic: A drug that affects the brain, often via the stomach and its nerves, it may be either sedative or stimulant. Sedative narcotics, such as OPIUM, inhibit nervous activity, promote sleep, and relieve pain, without causing sensible evacuations (e.g., sweat or stools). Stimulant narcotics, such as BELLADONNA, stimulate the mind and increase some evacuations, muscle activity, and the frequency and force of the pulse.

NARCOTICUS AETHIOPICUS: Same as AETHIOPS NARCOTICUS.

NARD, INDIAN: See NARDUS INDICA.

NARDUS INDICA: Root of Indian nard, or spikenard, *Nar-*

dostachys jatamansi. Stomachic, carminative, alexipharmic, diuretic, and emmenagogue. [15]

Nasalia: Errhines.

NASTURTIUM AQUATICUM: Leaves of watercress, *Nasturtium officinale*. Aperient and antiscorbutic. [15]

NATRON (or NATRUM): Same as BARILLA.

NEAPOLITAN OPIATE: Made with SENNA, SARSAPARILLA, SASSAFRAS, HERMODACTYLUS, and honey (but not OPIUM). Sedative.

NEAPOLITAN UNGUENT: A MERCURIAL ointment for skin disorders, especially syphilis and itch. [2]

NEAT FOOT OIL: See OLEUM BUBULUM.

NEPENTHES: Same as LAUDANUM.

NEPETA: Leaves of catnip, *Nepeta cataria*. Tonic, antispasmodic, and emmenagogue; also used as a toothache remedy. [15,29]

Nephritic: A remedy for disordered kidneys; a diuretic.

NEPHRITICA, AQUA: Spirit of NUTMEG with hawthorn (*Crataegus* spp.) flowers. For urinary disorders. [15]

NEPHRITICOS, DECOCTUM AD: A complex mixture of which the chief ingredient was ALTHAEA; it also included CARICA, LINI, GLYCERRHIZA, DAUCUS SYLVESTRIS, and root of the restharrow, or cammock (*Ononis arvensis*), a common field shrub. Used for renal colic. [15]

NEPHRITICUM LIGNUM: "Nephritic wood," probably the South American sp. *Guilandina moringa*, first described by Dr. Nicolas Monardes of Seville in 1565. The wood was made into a cup that turned water allowed to stand in it a deep blue. Diuretic, for renal disorders. [15]

Nervine: 1) In the 17th century, an emollient unguent for the sinews. 2) From the 18th century, a stimulating tonic for weak nerves.

NERVINUM, UNGUENTUM: "Nervine ointment." A mixture of OLEUM BUBULUM, VINUM, and OL TEREBINTHA, it was later modified as UNGUENTUM LAURINUM. Tonic; emollient. [2]

NETTLE, COMMON: See URTICA.

NEUTRAL MIXTURE: Same as LIQUOR POTASSAE CITRATIS.

NICOLAI, REQUIES: See REQUIES NICOLAI.

NICOTIANA [TABACUM]: Leaves of tobacco, *Nicotiana tabacum*. Introduced from the New World to Europe by

Spanish explorers shortly after 1492, it entered medical practice soon after French diplomat Jean Nicot described its medical effects in 1559, three years after André Thévet brought the first tobacco to Europe. Narcotic, emetic, diaphoretic, and diuretic; used powdered as an errhine (i.e., as snuff), or as a cutaneous insecticide; cathartic and anthelminthic when given as an enema or by fumigation. The essential oil is highly toxic. [2,15,23,29,30] Dried tobacco leaf contains about 6% nicotine, which was isolated by German chemists Christian Wilhelm Posselt and Karl Ludwig Reiman in 1828.

NICOTIANA, VIN: NICOTIANA steeped in white wine. Administered as a quick-acting diuretic, occasionally as an expectorant or mild laxative; given, rarely, per rectum for severe constipation, but too dangerous for routine use in this way. Also see SNUFF. [1,2]

NIGELLA: Roots of goldthread, *Coptis groenlandica*. Tonic, astringent, and digestive. [23,29,30]

NIGHTSHADE: See BELLADONNA and DULCAMARA.

NIGHTSHADE, AMERICAN: Same as PHYTOLACCA DECANDRA.

NITER (or NITRE), [SAL]: Potassium nitrate, saltpeter. Refrigerant, diuretic, resolvent, antiseptic, mild cathartic, and diaphoretic (but suppresses sweating when the pulse is slow and weak). Contraindicated in hemorrhage and bilious fevers. Side effects include vomiting, convulsions, and colic. [1,2,15,23,29].

NITER, [GLAUBER'S] SPIRIT OF: Nitrous acid, HNO_2, made by mixing SAL NITER with VITRIOL. Introduced by Dr. Johann Rudolph Glauber of Amsterdam about 1650. Cathartic and diuretic; also used as a fumigant to destroy contagion. [2,23]

NITRAS: A salt of ACIDUM NITRICUM.

NITRAS ARGENTI: Same as ARGENTUM NITRATUM.

NITRAS POTASSAE: Same as SAL NITER.

NITRATUM, ARGENTUM: See ARGENTUM NITRATUM.

NITRICUM, ACIDUM: Nitric acid, HNO_3. Antiphlogistic, tonic, antiseptic, and antisyphilitic. [23,29]

NITRITI, or NITRI, SAL: Same as SAL NITER.

NITRITI, UNGUENTUM: Antiseptic wound ointment made with SAL NITER. [1]

NITROSI, SPIRITUS AETHERIS: Same as DULCIFIED SPIRITS OF NITRE.

NITROSUM, ACIDUM: Same as SPIRIT OF NITER.

NITROUS OXIDE: Discovered by Rev. Joseph Priestley in 1772; Humphrey Davy uncovered its anesthetic properties in 1798, and Dr. Thomas Beddoes administered it to pulmonary disease patients a year later. Although its clinical anesthetic value was demonstrated in London in 1800, and in the U.S. by lecturer Dr. Horace Wells in 1844, its use in dentistry was popularized by itinerant chemistry lecturer Dr. Gardner Q. Colton only in 1863.

NITRUM: Same as SAL NITER.

NITRUM STIBIATUM: Same as ANTIMONIUM CALCINATUM.

NOUFFER'S (or NUFFER'S) TAPEWORM CURE: Powdered FILIX, the major drug administered during a 3-4 day treatment for tapeworms first reported by Mme. Nouffer, widow of a Swiss surgeon, in 1775. [13] However, Bigelow supposed that she added some true cathartics to insure that her remedy would be efficacious. [30, p. 296; for the full Nouffer treatment, see ref. 27, pp. 667-668]

NUREMBERG CERATE: A plaster made with OL ROSMARINUS, CAMPHOR, and MINIUM. Astringent and resolvent.

NUTMEG (and MACE): Seed of *Myristica fragrans*; mace is the dried external seed coat. Aromatic tonic, narcotic, stomachic, antiemetic, and astringent (but mace is less potent than nutmeg). Overdose produces stupor, delirium, and death. [2,15,23,29]

NUT OIL: Same as RICINI.

NUTRITUM, UNGUENTUM: "Nourishing ointment." Made with CERUSSA ACETATA.

NUX MOSCHATA [MARE]: Same as NUTMEG.

NUX PISTACHIA: Pistachio nut, *Pistachia vera*. Analeptic. [15]

NUX VOMICA: Literally, "ulcerated nut," because one side of the oblate seed has a depressed center. Dog-button, the seed of *Strychnos nux-vomica*. Introduced from southeast Asia, it was known to German medicine by 1540, but was reintroduced to modern medicine by Dr. François Magendie in 1821. In small doses, said to be tonic, diuretic, and sometimes diaphoretic and cathartic, and therefore appropriate for treating some fevers, including dysentery. In larger doses, "its [narcotic] action appears to be directed chiefly to the nerves of motion, probably through the medium of the spinal marrow," resulting in rigidity, spasms, convulsions, and death in respiratory failure. A bitter tonic, a narcotic, and a specific for the bite of a water snake. [15,29,30] French chemists Pierre-Joseph Pelletier and Joseph-Bienaimée Caventou isolated the potent alkaloid convulsants strychnine (1.0-1.4%) and brucine (which is less potent) from dog-buttons, ST. IGNATIUS'S BEANS, and other species in 1818-24. Strychnine is now used only as a pesticide.

NYMPHAEA ALBA: Root and flowers of white water lily, *Nymphaea* spp. Astringent; occasionally said to be narcotic. [15]

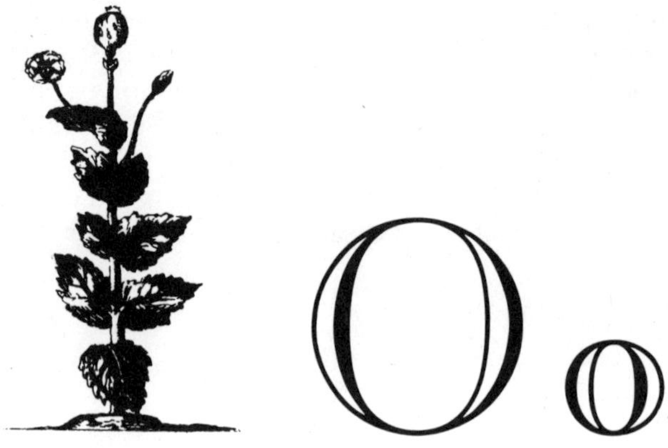

Opium

OAK: See QUERCUS entries.

OATS: See AVENA.

OCHRA: Yellow ochre, yellowish iron oxides, $FeO(OH) \cdot nH_2O$. Its properties are those of FERRUM. [15]

Octarius: Pint; see Measurement.

OCULI CANCRORUM: Same as CANCRORUM LAPILLI.

Odontalgica: Toothache remedies.

Odontites: Toothache remedies.

Odontotrimma: Remedies that clean and strengthen the teeth.

OENANTHE: Roots and leaves of the hemlock dropwort, or water hemlock, *Oenanthe fistulosa* or *O. crocata*. Antiscorbutic. Long known as "a most violent poison," it produces severe vomiting, convulsions, delirium, "and other terrible affections of the nervous system." [15] Contains an alkaloid that produces effects like those of coniine; see CICUTA.

Ointment: Same as Unguentum.

OINTMENT, SIMPLE: OL OLIVA, five parts, and CERA ALBA, two parts; cf. SIMPLE LINIMENT. [2]

Ol, or Oleum: An oil or an oily drug.

OLEA EUROPEA: Same as OL OLIVA.

OLEOSA SIMPLEX, EMULSIO: "Simple oily emulsion." A gargle made with OL AMYGDALA, ALTHAEA, GUM ARABIC. For sore throats. [1,15]

OLEOSA VOLATILIS, EMULSIO: "Volatile oily emulsion." Same as EMULSIO OLEOSA SIMPLEX, but with SPIRITUS AMMONIAE added to minimize the side effects of the OL AMYGDALA.

OLIBANUM: Frankincense, the gum resin of *Boswellia carteri*. Stimulant diaphoretic and cathartic. [15] By the mid-19th century, used chiefly only for fumigations and in some plasters. [29]

OLIVA, OL: Olive oil, expressed from the fruit of *Oliva europaea*. A demulcent used in plasters, ointments, and enemas; in emulsions, conserves, and linctuses for sore throat and cough; in cathartic medicines; in anthelminthics; and as an antidote to rattlesnake venom. [2,15,23,29,30] Its chief constituent is olein, or triolein.

OMOTRIBES: Oil expressed from hard green olives.

OMPHACINUM, OLEUM: Same as OMOTRIBES.

ONION: Same as CEPA.

OPHTHALMIA, AQUA: An aqueous collyrium.

OPHTHALMIC UNGUENT: Same as UNGUENT TUTIAE, or, sometimes, BAUME DE FIORAVANTI. [2]

OPIATA, CONFECTIO: A relatively weak opiate derived from earlier formulas for THERIACA ANDROMACHI; made with OPIUM, PIPER LONGUM, ZINGIBER, CARUON, and syrup of PAPAVER ALBUM.

OPIATUM, ELECTUARIUM: A relatively weak opiate derived from earlier formulas for THERIACA ANDROMACHI; made with 3 drachms OPIUM, 6 oz. PULVIS AROMATICUS, and 3 oz. SERPENTINA.

OPIATUM, LINIMENTUM [or UNGUENTUM]: A mixture of OPIUM, CAMPHOR, WINE, OL ROSMARINUS, and SAPO. Used most often as a topical analgesic, but sometimes internally. [2,15,23]

OPIATUS, PULVIS: A mixture of OPIUM and CRETA.

OPII AMMONIATA, TINCTURA: "Ammoniated tincture of opium," made with OPIUM, FLOWERS OF BENZOIN, SAFFRON, ANISUM, and SPIRITUS AMMONIAE. Used for all indications for OPIUM. [15]

OPII CAMPHORATA, TINCTURA: "Camphorated tincture of opium." Alcohol extract of OPIUM, CAMPHOR, BENZOIN, and ANISUM; nearly same as PAREGORIC.

Used for all indications for OPIUM, and especially as an antitussive (hence its frequent synonym Elixir Asthmaticus). [15] The same ingredients are in modern paregoric.

OPII QUERCETANI, EXTRACTUM: Same as QUERCETANUS'S EXTRACT OF OPIUM.

OPIUM: Dried latex exudate of seed pods of opium poppy, *Papaver somniferum.* Because it decreases the irritability of most tissues and organs, opium is a sedative narcotic, appropriately prescribed as a sedative, soporific, analgesic, antitussive, antispasmodic, and antidiarrheal, and to relax the common bile duct when obstructed by a stone. It is sometimes given with CALOMEL to ameliorate active inflammatory processes, especially those producing pain and fever, such as septic wounds, by diverting the "morbid action" away from the site of inflammation, or to neutralize the effects of cathartics. When taken internally, opium induces serenity and drowsiness, slows the pulse, dilates the veins, causes sweating, and reduces bowel discharge by inhibiting intestinal muscle activity. Since this constipating effect often counteracts therapeutic cathartics, opium is sometimes used alone as an antidiarrheal. Large doses induce confusion, vertigo, and deep sleep, while even larger doses produce tremors, delirium, convulsions, stupor, dyspnea, and coma (opium-induced death was associated with respiratory failure by the early 19th century). The adverse effects of opium include constipation, addiction, and, in some people, an idiosyncratic reaction characterized by nausea and vomiting, and headache with delirium. Finally, patients may fail to respond to previously effective doses, because "Habitual use renders the system unsusceptible of the original effect," necessitating large increases in dose to allay chronic pains (this correctly describes the phenomenon now called tolerance). On the other hand, pain can antagonize opium's narcotic effect. [1,2,3,15,23,29,30] It seems odd that miosis (pin-point pupils) was not recognized as a regular effect of opium until 1818. Several drugs that contained no opium were called opiates only because they were as sticky as raw opium (e.g., NEAPOLITAN OPIATE). Raw opium contains 10-20% morphine, isolated in 1806 (although published only in 1817) by Friedrich Wilhelm Sertürner, of Paderborn, Westphalia, and 0.3-4.0% codeine, isolated in 1832 by French chemist Pierre Jean Robiquet, and about 23 other related alkaloids. As early as 1827 Heinrich Emanuel Merck of Darmstadt began to manufacture morphine in a form suitable for injection from an eye syringe through a cut in the skin. The chief tools for administering morphine today, the hypodermic needle and syringe, which permit administering very precise doses, were invented in 1853, but oral preparations are becoming increasingly popular again.

OPIUM ENEMA: OPIUM added to DOMESTIC ENEMA. A potent inhibitor of gastrointestinal activity for treating both vomiting and diarrhea, it also produces analgesia and sedation. [1,2,3,15]

OPIUM, PILL OF: Usually, but not necessarily, same as THEBAIC PILL.

OPIUM, TINCTURE OF: Same as LAUDANUM, PAREGORIC, or TINCTURA THEBAICA.

OPOBALSAMUM: Same as BALM OF GILEAD.

OPODELDOC: A word applied by Paracelsus to certain plasters, but it had become a proprietary soap liniment by the 18th century. An early American version was made with OL ROSMARINUS, OL MENTHA, CAMPHORA, AQUA AMMONIAE, ALCOHOL, and soap. See STEER'S OPODELDOC for a later version. [14]

OPOPANAX: 1) Gum resin of root of *Opopanax chironium*. Gentle cathartic, deobstruent, antispasmodic, and emmenagogue. [15,29] 2) Juice of LIGUSTICUM.

ORANGE: Usually the peel; see CORTEX AURANTIUM.

ORCHID (or ORCHIS [MASCULA]): See SATYRION.

OREGANO: See ORIGANUM.

ORIGANUM: Wild majoram, now usually called oregano, *Origanum vulgare*. Aromatic with little specific medicinal use, but said to be errhine, tonic, diaphoretic, emmenagogue, and a dental analgesic. [15,29]

ORIGANUM MAJORANA: Same as MAJORANA.

ORPIMENT: Lemon-yellow arsenic trisulfide, As_2S_3.

ORRIS ROOT: Samc as IRIS FLORENTINA.

ORVIETANUM: An antidote containing OPIUM; named for the town in Italy where it was invented.

ORYZA: Grains of rice, *Oryza sativa*. Nutritious, a "useful food" in diarrhea. [15]

OSTREA EDULIS: Pulverized shells of oyster, *Ostrea* spp. Antacid; sometimes burned to make QUICKLIME.

Ounce [Oz.]: See Measurement.

OVI, OL: Egg oil, expressed from hard-boiled eggs that have been broken and fried. Antidiarrheal and styptic. [15]

OVIS [ARIES], or SEVUM OVILLUM: Mutton suet, used as a lubricating and relaxing ointment, as a diaphoretic, and for compounding several ointments, liniments, and plasters. [15]

OVUM: Egg of hen, *Gallus gallus*. Both whites and yolks were used to give appropriate consistency to several medicines. Shells were sometimes burned to make QUICKLIME, or used, after pulverizing, as an antacid. Egg whites were used as an antidote for poisoning with copper or mercury salts, or to make poultices, while the yolk was sometimes employed as a cathartic, especially, because of its color, in jaundice. [15,29]

OXALIS [ACETOSA]: Same as ACETOSA.

OXALIS ACETOSELLA: Same as LUJULA.

OXIDUM ANTIMONII: Same as CROCUS ANTIMONII.

OXIDUM ANTIMONII CUM SULPHURETUM, PER NITRATEM POTASSAE: Same as CROCUS ANTIMONII.

OXIDUM ANTIMONII VITRIFICATUM, CUM CERA: Same as ANTIMONII VITRUM CERATUM.

OXIDUM ANTIMONIUM CUM PHOSPHATE CALCIS: Same as PULVIS ANTIMONIALIS.

OXIDUM ANTIMONIUM, CUM SULPHURE, VITRIFICATUM: Same as ANTIMONIUM VITRIFICATUM.

OXIDUM ARSENICI: Sames as WHITE ARSENIC.

OXIDUM FERRI NIGRUM PURIFICATUM: Black oxide of iron, or iron scales; essentially same as FERRI LIMATURA PURIFICATA.

OXIDUM FERRI RUBRUM: Same as FERRI RUBIGO.

OXIDUM HYDRARGYRI CINEREUM: Same as HYDRARGYRUS PRAECIPITATUS.

OXIDUM HYDRARGYRI ET AMMONIAE: Same as WHITE PRECIPITATE.

OXIDUM HYDRARGYRI RUBRUM: Same as HYDRARGYRUS NITRATUS RUBER.

OXIDUM PLUMBI ALBUM: Same as WHITE LEAD.

OXIDUM PLUMBI RUBRUM: Same as RED LEAD.

OXIDUM PLUMBI SEMIVITREUM: Same as WHITE LEAD, but rendered semi-crystalline by heat.

OXIDUM ZINCI [IMPURUM]: Same as ZINCUM USTUM.

OXYCANTHA GALENI: Same as BERBERIS.

Oxycoos: A remedy for earache.

Oxycratum: A mixture including ACETUM and water.

OXYCRATUM SATURNI: Same as LAC VIRGINAL, def. no. 1.

OXYCROCEUM, EMPLASTRUM: "Saffron plaster," made with CROCUS, PIX BURGUNDICA, CERA FLAVA, GALBANUM, and PIX LIQUIDA.

Oxyfragium: Any alkaline antacid remedy.

OXYLAPATHUM: Same as HYDROLAPATHUM.

Oxymel: A preparation in which the active drug ingredient was mixed with vinegar and honey.

OXYMEL SIMPLEX: A drink made of vinegar and honey. [2,15] Expectorant.

Oxyporion: A penetrating remedy, e.g., RHAMNUS CATHARTICUS.

OXYRHODINUM: Oil of ROSES and ACETUM.

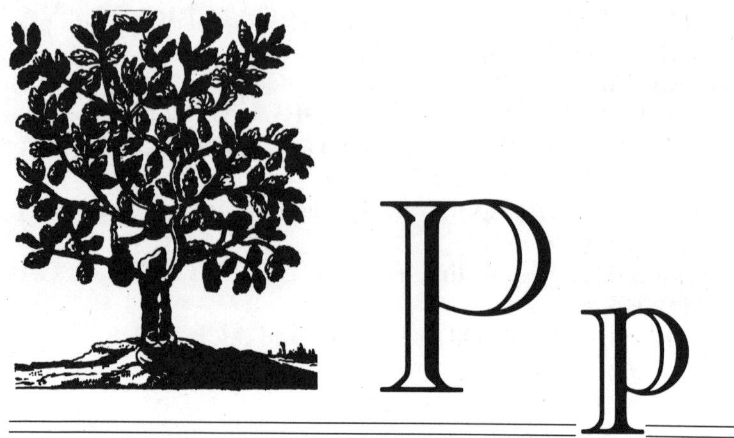

Peru, Balsam of

PACIFICK PILL, DR. BATE'S: A preparation devised in the mid-17th century by Dr. William Bate of London, it contained about 30% OPIUM, or 1.0-5.9 mg. morphine per recommended dose, depending on body weight, as well as CROCUS, ACIDUM TARTARICUM, ANETHUM, and soap. [3]

PACIFIC PILL: Same as THEBAIC PILL, with added PIMENTO.

PAEONIA: Root and seed of peonies, *Paeonia* spp. (supposedly named for Paion, physician to the Greek gods). Emollient, corroborant, deobstruent, and slightly anodyne, but especially antispasmodic and antiepileptic. [15]

Palliativa Remedia: Remedies that mitigate pain without removing its cause, e.g., OPIUM.

PALMA: Oil of unspecified palm trees. Used in external remedies, especially antirheumatic liniments. [15,23]

PALMAE CHRISTI, OLEUM: "Oil of palm of Christ," same as castor oil; see RICINI.

PALMA, WHITE POWDER OF THE COUNT OF: Same as MAGNESIA ALBA.

PALSY DROPS: Same as COMPOUND SPIRITS OF LAVENDER.

Panacea: A cure-all. (There is no evidence that a mythological Panacea was a daughter of Aesculapius.)

PANACEA ANTIMONIALIS (or ANTIMONII): "Antimony panacea." 1) An evaporated mixture of SAL TARTARI and ANTIMONIUM MURIATUM. 2) A mixture of ANTIMONIUM, SAL NITER, SAL MURIATICUS, and PULVIS CARBONAS LIGNI. Both formulations are cathartic and emetic. [15]

PANACEA CINNABARINA SIVE MERCURIUS DIAPHORETICUS: "Cinnabar panacea, or diaphoretic mercury." Same as THOMPSON'S PANACEA.

PANACEA HOLSATICA: Literally, "Sea–kale [*Crambe maritima*, formerly *Smyrnium holusatrum*] panacea." Same as KALI SULPHURATUM.

PANACEA, LIQUID: An aquaeous preparation containing 20-25% OPIUM; 20 drops produced the same effect as 1 gr. SOLID PANACEA. [3]

PANACEA MERCURIALIS: "Mercurial panacea," multiply recrystallized CALOMEL in SPIRITUS VINOSUS.

PANACEA MERCURIALIS VIOLACEA: "Violet mercurial panacea." CALOMEL mixed with SULPHUR and SAL AMMONIAC.

PANACEA, SOLID: A strong OPIUM and soap pill containing 3.3-13.0 mg. morphine per recommended dose, depending on body weight. [3]

PANADA (or PANADO): Bread boiled to a pulp in water and flavored to taste.

PANAROLIS'S MEDICINE: An ointment devised about 1650 by Dr. Domenico Panarolis of Rome, it was made with SULPHUR and SUCCUS LIMONI in lard.

PANAX: Same as GINSENG.

Panchymagoga: Remedies that purge all the humors.

Pancrestum: A panacea.

PANDALEON: A pectoral electuary made with OPIUM.

Panis Parvus: "Small bread," a troche.

PANIS REGIUS: "Royal bread," a cordial, stomachic, and pectoral electuary.

PAPALIS, CONFECTIO: "Papal confection." Tablets of ALTHAEA.

PAPAVER ALBUM: Extract of seed pod (not the resinous

exudate, although it was surely inside the pod) of the white poppy strain of *Papaver somniferum*; because it is only about one-half as potent as OPIUM, it is deemed especially suitable for children. [15] Poppy heads contain about 0.7% morphine when fresh, and less as they ripen.

PAPAVER ERRATICUM (or RHOEAS): Juice of flowers of red poppy, *Papaver rhoeas*. Only slightly analgesic; used chiefly for its color. [15,29]

PAPAVER SOMNIFERUM: Same as OPIUM.

PARACELSI, EMPLASTRUM: "Plaster of Paracelsus," probably same as DIACHYLON, which evolved from the SYMPATHETIC UNGUENT OF PARACELSUS. [2]

PARACELSI, SPECIFICUM PURGANS: "Specific purgative of Paracelsus," same as KALI SUPLPHURATUM.

PAREGORIC [ELIXIR]: Tincture of 0.2% OPIUM as well as BENZOIN, CAMPHOR, GLYCERRHIZA, OL ANISUM, and MEL DESPUMATUM, but also see TINCTURA OPII CAMPHORATA. The adjective "paregoric" means "soothing." Narcotic, antitussive, and antidiarrheal. [2,15]

PAREIRA BRAVA: Root of the South American vine *Chondrodendron tomentosum*. Introduced to Lisbon from Brazil in the 17th century, and to Paris in 1688. Tonic, aperient, diuretic, and expectorant; sometimes used as a lithontriptic. [15,29] Although no orally active materials have been isolated from this plant, it is the source of the muscle relaxant curare (which must be administered parenterally to produce muscle paralysis). Curare's use as an arrow poison in South America was first noted in 1516 (by Pietro Martire d'Anghiera). Although the mechanism of curare's paralytic action was studied experimentally in the 18th and early 19th centuries, it was elucidated, by Claude Bernard, only in 1857. The neuromuscular (nicotinic) blocking activity of curare became a valuable adjunct to surgical anesthia only after 1940.

PAREITARIA: Pellitory of the wall, *Parietaria officinalis*, *P. erecta*, or *P. diffusa*. Emollient and diuretic. [15] Contains potassium nitrate, i.e., NITER.

Pargyron: 1) A liquid medicine. 2) A plaster.

PARSLEY: See PETROSELINUM.

PARSNIP: See PASTINACA.

PARSNIP, WATER: See SIUM.

PASQUEFLOWER: See PULSATILLA NIGRICANS.

Pastille: An aromatic or perfumed troche.

PASTINACA: Seeds of parsnips, *Pastinaca sativa*. Aromatic.

PEACH: See PERSICA.

PEARL ASH: Same as LIXIVA.

PEARL BARLEY: Same as HORDEUM PERLATUM.

Pectoral: A remedy for disorders of the chest and lungs, with antitussive and expectorant properties.

Pedilave: Same as Pediluvium.

Pediluvium: A decoction for bathing the feet and legs in drugs appropriate to the patient's illness.

PELLEGRIN, LIQUEUR DE: See LIQUEUR DE PELLEGRIN.

PELLITORY, BASTARD or WILD: See PTARMICA.

PELLITORY OF THE WALL: See PAREITARIA.

PELLITORY, SPANISH: See PYRETHRUM.

PENIDIA: Same as SACCHARUM PENIDIATUM.

PENIS SYRINGE: A syringe used for intra-urethral injections.

PENNYROYAL: See PULEGIUM.

PENTAPHYLLUM: Root of cinquefoil, *Potentilla reptans*. Weak astringent. [15]

PEONY: See PAEONIA.

PEPPER: See PIMENTO and PIPER.

PEPPER, BLACK: See PIPER NIGRUM.

PEPPER, CAYENNE (or GUINEA): See PIPER INDICUM.

PEPPER, JAMAICA: See PIMENTO.

PEPPER, LONG: See PIPER LONGUM.

PEPPERMINT: See MENTHA PIPERITA and ESSENCE OF PEPPERMINT.

PEPPER, WATER: See PERSICARIA.

Peptic powder, pill, etc.: A medicine that stimulates digestion in the stomach; usually contains tonic drugs. [2]

PERKINS' TRACTORS: A pair of metallic spikes patented by Dr. Elisha Perkins of Connecticut (1740-1799) in 1796. He promoted them for removing pains and inflammations from the body by drawing them over the body surface. Perkins said that one tractor was made of copper, zinc, and a bit of gold, and the other of iron with traces of silver and platinum, but a contemporary chemical analysis showed the first to be made of brass and the second of iron. Although the tractors have been perceived by some as quackery, that is too harsh a judgment on Perkins's professional motives. [Jacques M.

Quen, "Elisha Perkins, Physician, Nostrum Vendor, or Charlatan?," *Bulletin of the History of Medicine 37* (1963): 159-166; and any edition of Oliver Wendell Holmes's essay on "Homeopathy and its Kindred Delusions"]

PERPETUA, PILULE: A pill made of ANTIMONIUM, SAL TARTARI, and SAL NITER, to promote prolonged catharsis.

PERSICA: Flowers, seeds, and leaves of the peach, *Prunus persica*. Mild cathartic, sedative, and anthelminthic. [15]

PERSICARIA: Leaves of the water-pepper, or smartweed, *Polygonum hydropiper*. Tonic diuretic, antiscorbutic, and discutient. [15]

PERSIMMON: See DIOSPYROS.

PERU, APPLE OF: Same as STRAMONIUM.

PERU, BALSAM OF: Extract of *Myroxylon pereirae*. Introduced from Central America to Spain about 1525 (should not be confused with Peruvian Bark, CINCHONA). Tonic, attenuant, emmenagogue, expectorant, and vulnerary. [2,15,23,29]

PERU, RHUBARB OF: Same as MECHOACANNA.

PERUVIAN BARK: Same as CINCHONA.

Pessary: A medicated substance, usually an antihysteric, for insertion into the vagina.

PETASITIS: Root of the butterbur, *Petasites vulgaris*. Aperient, deobstruent, and aromatic. [15]

PETER, OIL OF: "Rock oil," same as PETROLEUM.

PETER'S PILLS: A 19th-century proprietary cathartic made with ALOES, CALOMEL, GAMBOGE, JALAP, and SCAMMONIUM.

PETROLEUM [BARBADENSE]: Literally, "rock oil." Mineral, or fossil oils, and their distillates; the Barbadoes product was thicker than others. Described in 1629 by Franciscan friar De la Roche D'Allia. A stimulating antispasmodic used chiefly as a liniment, but also, rarely, as a mild cathartic, diaphoretic, anthelminthic, and expectorant when ingested. [23,29]

PETROLEUM SULPHURATUM: Same as OLEUM SULPHURATUM.

PETROSELINUM: Root and seed of parsley, *Petroselinum crispum*. Used in apozemata and diet drinks as a carminative, aperient, and diuretic; also an emmenagogue. [15]

PHAGEDENIC WATER: "Ulcer water." Aqueous solution of CALOMEL, for skin inflammations, ulcers, and chancres.

Pheonigmus: Same as a SINAPISM.

PHILONIUM PERSICUM: "Persian medicine." A preparation containing 5.7% OPIUM, providing 5.9-22.2 mg. morphine per recommended dose, depending on body weight, as well as PIPER ALBUM, HELLEBORUS ALBUS, LEMNIAN EARTH, HEMATITE, CROCUS, CAMPHORA, CONSERVE OF ROSES, and nine aromatics. [3,13]

PHILONIUM ROMANUM: "Roman medicine." A preparation containing about 2.5% OPIUM, which provided 2.6-9.8 mg. morphine per recommended dose, depending on body weight, as well as PIPER NIGRUM, HELLEBORUS ALBUS, CASSIA LIGNEA, PETROSELINUM, FOENICULUM DULCE, DAUCUS CRETICUS, CROCUS, MEL DESPUMATUM, and six aromatics. [3,13]

PHILOSOPHORUM, OLEUM: "Philosophers' oil." Medieval alchemists' name for what was later sold as BRITISH OIL.

Phlegmagoga: Remedies that purge the pituitary gland and, therefore, the throat, of phlegm.

PHOENIX DACTYLIFERA: See DACTYLUS.

PHOSPHAS CALCIS: Same as HARTSHORN.

PHOSPHAS SODAE: Same as SODA PHOSPHORATA.

PHOSPHATE MIXTURE: Mixture of HARTSHORN and SODA PHOSPHORATA. For rickets. [2]

PHOSPHORATED SODA: Same as SODA PHOSPHORATA.

PHOSPHORICUM, ACIDUM: Phosphoric acid, isolated from bones by Angelo Sala in Germany about 1637. Tonic, refrigerant, analgesic, antispasmodic, aphrodisiac, and antilithic. [29]

PHOSPHORUS: Discovered in Hamburg in 1669, and identified in bones by Gahn in 1769. Because phosphorus emits light (even if it does not produce heat), it was interpreted as a chemical analogue of combustion and respiration, and, therefore, as a tonic agent. In small doses, a potent general stimulant; in large doses, a violent irritant poison. Produces diuresis, excites the libido, and stimulates weak nerves. [29,30]

Phthartica: Fatal poisons.

Phthoria: Remedies that hasten childbirth.

Phthoropoeum: A poison.

PHYSETER MACROCEPHALUS: Same as SPERMACETI.

Physogonum: A carminative.

PHYTOLACCA DECANDRA: Berries, leaves, and roots of pokeweed, garget, or American nightshade, *Phytolacca decandra*. Slow-acting emetic; cathartic; somewhat narcotic; can substitute for GUIAC. [23,29,30]

Picatio: A depilatory plaster; see, e.g., EMPLASTRUM PICEUM.

PICEAE, PILULE: "Tar pill," made with PIX LIQUIDA and ENULA CAMPANA.

PICEUM, EMPLASTRUM: "Tar plaster," made with PIX LIQUIDA or PIX BURGUNDICA. When applied externally, tar has both warming and adhesive properties; hence it is used for tinea capitis because it removes the hair bulbs when the plaster is removed.

PICIS BURGUNDICAE COMPOSITUM, EMPLASTRUM: "Compound plaster of Burgundy pitch." Made with PIX BURGUNDICA, LADANUM, OL MACIS, OL TEREBINTHA, and CERA FLAVA. Rubefacient and vesicant; used for headaches. [15]

PIERMONT WATER: A mineral water from Pyrmont, near Hanover, Germany. Regarded as a tonic because it is rich in FERRI RUBIGO, it also contained the cathartic salts MAGNESIA ALBA, MAGNESIA VITRIOLATA, and SAL MURIATICUS. [20,46]

PILEWORT: See CHELIDONIUM MINUS.

PILL UNIQUE: A proprietary medicine containing mercury and antimony. Cathartic. [2]

Pilule: A pill, a dosage form used to maximize the duration of a drug's action compared with liquid formulations. Made with gummy resins, soap, inspissated juices, syrup, honey, and other binding agents.

PIMENTO (or PIMENTA): Berries of pimento, also called allspice and Jamaica pepper, *Pimenta officinalis*. Introduced to Europe from the West Indies about 1600, and to medical practice soon after. Used as a cordial tonic and carminative, chiefly in julaps and draughts. [15,23,29]

PIMPERNEL: See ANAGALLIS.

PIMPINELLA: Root of burnet saxifrage, *Pimpinella saxifraga*. Emollient, stomachic, resolvent, detergent, expectorant, diuretic, diaphoretic, febrifuge, alexipharmic, and antiscorbutic. [15]

PIMPINELLA ANISUM: Same as ANISUM.

PINE: See ABIETES, PIX LIQUIDA, and TEREBINTHA.

PINK, or PINKROOT: See SPIGELIA.

PINKROOT, CAROLINA: See SPIGELIA.

Pint: See Measurement.

PINUS ABIES: Same as BALSAMUM CANADENSE.

PINUS BALSAMEA: Probably same as PINUS ABIES.

PINUS LARIX: Larch tree, *Larix decidua* (and other spp.), a source of OL TEREBINTHA.

PINUS SYLVESTRIS: Scotch pine, *Pinus sylvestris*, a source of PIX LIQUIDA.

PIPER ALBA: White pepper; see PIPER NIGRUM.

PIPER INDICUM: Fruit of a variety of Cayenne pepper, *Capsicum frutescens* (however, it was often adulterated with other species). Stimulant and digestive. [15,29]

PIPER LONGUM: Fruit or distilled oil of the long pepper, *Piper longum*, the strongest of all hot peppers. Introduced to Europe from East Indies by 1550s. [15]

PIPER NIGRUM: Ground whole berry, or its distilled oil, of black pepper, *Piper nigrum* (white pepper is the ground seed, after removal of the black shells). Aromatic and stimulating digestive; also used to control nausea, vomiting, and hiccups. [15,23,29]

PIPSISSEWA: See CHIMAPHILA.

PISTACHIA: See MASTICHE and NUX PISTACHIA.

PITCH, or PIX: Tar.

PIX ABIETIS: Same as PIX BURGUNDICA.

PIX BURGUNDICA: Burgundy pitch, resin of spruce fir, *Abies excelsa*, or *A. balsamea* (also see BALSAMUM CANADENSE), but other spp. or just TEREBINTHA were sometimes sold as such. Used chiefly only in ointments and plasters, as a rubefacient. [15,23,29]

PIX CANADENSIS: Same as BALSAMUM CANADENSIS.

PIX LIQUIDA: Tar, or oil distilled from roots of PINUS SYLVESTRIS, and other species. Warm, stimulating expectorant. [15,23,29]

PIX NIGRA: Black pitch, the residue left after evaporation of PIX LIQUIDA. Gentle tonic, used internally, and externally for skin diseases. [29]

Placentula: A flat, round troche.

PLANTAGO: Leaves of common great plantain, *Plantago ma-*

jor. Astringent; also said to cure rattlesnake and venomous spider bites. [15,23]

PLANTAINS: See PLANTAGO, PSYLLIUM, and SATYRION.

Plaster: A powder mixed with an oily substance to a consistency that remains firm but pliable in the cold without sticking to the fingers, and which will adhere to both the skin on which it is applied and to the substance (e.g., linen cloth) on which it is spread.

PLENCK'S SOLUTION: See SOLUTIO MERCURIALIS SIMPLEX.

Pleonectica: Remedies that prevent accumulation of fluid in the body, e.g., hydragogue cathartics, diaphoretics, and diuretics.

PLERES ARCONTICON: A cephalic mixture.

PLEURISY ROOT: See ASCLEPIAS DECUMBENS.

PLUMBUM: Elemental lead. Its salts (e.g., CERUSSA ACETATA), taken internally, are sedative, astringent, incrassating, anti-inflammatory, and antaphrodisiac. Side effects of accidentally ingested or inhaled lead include severe colic, tremors, spasms, and palsy (paralysis). [15,23,30]

PLUMBUM ACETATUM: Same as CERUSSA ACETATA.

PLUMMER'S PILLS (or POWDER): A mixture of GOLDEN SULPHURET, CALOMEL, GENTIAN, and soap, described in 1733 by Dr. Andrew Plummer, professor of medicine at Edinburgh; later evolved into PILULE HYDRARGYROSI MURIATI MITIS.

PLUNKETT'S REMEDY: See ARSENICUM.

Pneumonica: Drugs that facilitate breathing.

POCULA EMETICA: "Emetic cup." Same as CUPPA EMETICA.

PODALYRIA TINCTORIA: "Dye of Podalirius [a son of Aesculapius]." Same as SOPHORA TINCTORIA.

PODOPHYLLUM PELTATUM: Root of may apple, or American mandrake, *Podophyllum peltatum*. First described by English naturalist Mark Catesby in 1731. Strong cathartic and anthelminthic; also emetic and antitussive. Side effects include severe dermatitis and conjunctivitis. [23,29,30] Its cathartic property is attributable to its ability to irritate the small intestine so as to inhibit the reaborption of water from the lumen. Its major alkaloid, podophyllotoxin, is sometimes used to remove benign skin growths, such as warts, and two of its derivatives (etoposide and teniposide) are used in the treatment of certain cancers.

POISON BERRY: Same as MELIA AZEDARACH.

POISON HEMLOCK: See CICUTA.

POISON IVY: See RHUS entries.

POKEROOT: 1) HELLEBORUS ALBUS. 2) PHYTOLACCA DECANDRA. 3) VERATRUM VIRIDE.

POKEWEED: Same as PHYTOLACCA DECANDRA.

Polyanodyna: Rapid-acting anodynes, e.g., OPIUM.

Polychrestum: A panacea; literally, "many virtues."

POLYCHRESTUM [POLYCHRIS] [GLASERI], BALSAM or SAL: "Salt of many virtues;" usually same as KALI SULPHURATUM, but sometimes MAGNESIA ALBA. Devised by Christopher Glaser, a Paracelsian French apothecary, in the 17th century. Cathartic. [2]

POLYCHRESTUM SEIGNETTE, SAL: See SEIGNETTE'S SALT.

POLYCHRESTUM STIBIALE, SAL: "Antimony panacea." A cathartic made with ANTIMONIUM.

POLYGALA SENEGA: Same as SENECA.

POLYGONATUM: See CONVALLARIA.

POLYGONUM BISTORTA: Same as BISTORTA.

POLYGONUM HYDROPIPER: See PERSICARIA.

POLYPODIUM: Root of polypody fern, *Polypodium vulgare*. Used to purge melancholy humors, or all the humors. Astringent, styptic, and antiscorbutic. [15]

POLYPODIUM FILIX MAS: Same as FILIX.

POMEGRANATE: See GRANATA MALUS.

POMPHOLYX: Impure zinc oxide; see ZINCUM USTUM.

POPLAR, AMERICAN: Same as LIRIODENDRON TULIPIFERA.

POPLAR, BLACK (or LOMBARDY): See POPULUS.

POPLAR, CAROLINA: See TACAMAHACA.

POPPY: See entries for OPIUM, PAPAVER ALBUM, and PAPAVER ERRATICUM; also see ARGEMONE MEXICANA.

POPULEUM, UNGUENTUM: "Poplar ointment," made with POPULUS, PAPAVER SOMNIFERUM leaves, MANDRAGORA, LACTUCA, BARDANA, VIOLA, etc., in AXUNGUENTUM PORCINUM. Febrifuge and soporific.

POPULUS: 1) Usually, buds of black or Lombardy poplar,

Populus nigra italica or other spp. Narcotic. [15] Contains populin, which is chemically like aspirin. 2) Sometimes, LIRIODENDRON TULIPIFERA.

PORRUM: Leek, *Allium porrum*. Stimulating diuretic. [29]

PORTER: Strong dark beer containing about 6.8% alcohol. Astringent tonic. [1]

PORTLAND, GOUT POWDER OF DUKE OF: An ancient remedy made of ARISTOLOCHIA, GENTIAN, CHAMAEDRYS, CHAMAEPITHYS, and CENTAURIUM MINUS that was resurrected by a mid-18th century English nobleman. [13]

Posca: An oxycratum.

Poscetum: Posset, milk curdled with beer, wine, or other liquor. A typical posset was a mixture of two parts of SMALL BEER and one part of milk (also see DIET).

POTASH: See LIXIVA.

POTASH, DRY: Same as POTASSAE, ACETIS.

POTASSAE, ACETIS: Potassium acetate. Diuretic and diaphoretic.

POTASSAE, AQUA: Potassium hydroxide solution. Lithontriptic when injected into the bladder via the urethra; antacid when ingested; caustic when applied topically. [23]

POTASSAE ARSENITIS, LIQUOR: Same as SOLUTIO MINERALIS ARSENICI.

POTASSAE BITARTRAS: Same as CREAM OF TARTAR.

POTASSAE CARBONAS IMPURUS: Same as LIXIVA.

POTASSAE CHLORAS: Potassium chloride. Refrigerant diuretic. [29]

POTASSAE CITRATIS, LIQUOR: Solution of potassium citrate in SODA WATER. Refrigerant diaphoretic and gastric sedative. [29]

POTASSAE NITRAS: Same as NITER.

POTASSAE SULPHAS: Same as KALI SULPHURATUM.

POTASSII BROMIDUM: Potassium bromide; discovered by French chemist Antoine-Jerôme Balard in 1826. Alterative and resolvent, when administered internally or externally. [29]

POTASSII FERROCYANURETUM: Potassium ferrocyanide. Sedative and anodyne. [29]

POTASSII IODIDUM: Potassium iodide. Stimulates all the secretions, especially saliva. Dr. James Copland, of the

Orkney Islands, introduced it for the treatment of syphilis because it had long been known to respond to HYDRARGYRUS, which also stimulates salivation. Side effects include skin eruptions. [29]

Poterium: A drink (literally, a drinking vessel).

Potus: A drink, or potion.

POTUS EXCITANS: A "stimulating drink" invented about 1800 by Dr. Joseph Frank of Pavia, Italy, as an especially Brunonian tonic. It was made with alcohol, honey, water, sugar, eggs, and nutmeg. [Guenter B. Risse, "Brunonian Therapeutics: New Wine in Old Bottles?," *Medical History* (1988), *Suppl. 8*, pp. 46-62]

POUNCE: Gum from JUNIPERUS COMMUNIS.

PRAECIPITATUM FLAVUM: "Yellow precipitate." Same as HYDRARGYRUS VITRIOLATUS FLAVUS.

PRECIPITE BLANC: See WHITE PRECIPITATE.

PRICKLY ASH: 1) Same as ARALIA SPINOSA. 2) In northern U.S., *Xanthoxylum fraxineum*. Stomachic, diaphoretic, and an antirheumatic anodyne. [30]

PRICKLY POPPY: Same as ARGEMONE MEXICANA.

PRIDE OF CHINA (or INDIA): Same as MELIA AZEDARACH.

PRINOS [VERTICILLATUS]: Bark and berries of winterberry, or black alder, *Ilex* spp. Bitter tonic and astringent. [23,29]

Prolifica: Aphrodisiacs.

PROOF SPIRIT: 100 proof (i.e., 50%) alcohol.

Prophylactica: Poison antidotes.

PROPHYLACTICUM, ACETUM: "Prophylactic vinegar." Same as ACETUM AROMATICUM.

PROPRIETATIS [PARACELSI], ELIXIR: "His [i.e., Paracelsus's] own elixir." Same as TINCTURA ALOES COMPOSITA.

PROTOCHLORIDE OF MERCURY: Same as CALOMEL.

PROTO-OXIDE OF AZOTE (or of NITRAS): Same as NITROUS OXIDE.

PRUNELLA: Self-heal, or heal-all, *Prunella vulgaris*. Vulnerary. [2,15]

PRUNELLAE, SAL: A red form of KALI SULPHURATUM devised by French Paracelsian apothecary Christopher Glaser about 1660, and named for its resemblance to PRUNUS SYLVESTRIS. Febrifuge.

PRUNUM: Same as PRUNUS GALLICA.

PRUNUS AMYGDALUS: See AMYGDALA entries.

PRUNUS CERASIFERA: See MYROBOLANS.

PRUNUS CERASUS [VIRGINIANA]: Same as CERASUS.

PRUNUS DOMESTICA: Same as PRUNUS GALLICA.

PRUNUS GALLICA: Common prune, *Prunus domestica*. Refrigerant and emollient cathartic. [15,23,29]

PRUNUS LAUROCERASUS: European cherry laurel, *Prunus laurocerasus*, the source of a poisonous oil resembling OL AMYGDALA. Native to northern Europe, but introduced to medicine only in 1731 following an epidemic of poisonings it had caused in Dublin. Narcotic; digestive. [23,29] The oil contains hydrocyanic acid, which had been identified by Swedish chemist Karl Wilhelm Scheele in 1782.

PRUNUS PERSICA: See PERSICA.

PRUNUS SYLVESTRIS: Fruit of blackthorn, or sloe, *Prunus spinosa*. Gentle astringent. [15]

PRUNUS VIRGINIANUS: Bark of wild black or choke cherry, *Prunus virginiana*. Introduced to medicine in the late 18th century, probably by American botanist John Bartram. Tonic, and calms the circulation, because of its hydrocyanic acid content. [29]

PRUSSIC ACID: Hydrocyanic acid. Although a potent poison, it was advocated as a sedative in the early 19th century. [30] See PRUNUS LAUROCERASUS.

Psilothrum: A depilatory.

Psorica: Remedies for itch.

Psyctica: Refrigerants.

PSYLLIUM: Seeds of fleawort, *Plantago psyllium*, a plantain spp. that yields a mucilage used in some emollient enemas. [15] Now thought to be antihypercholesterolemic.

PTARMICA: Roots or, sometimes, leaves, of sneezewort, or bastard or wild pellitory, *Achillea ptarmica*. Sialogogue; when powdered, used as an errhine. [15]

PTEROCARPI LIGNUM: Same as SANTALUM RUBRUM.

PTEROCARPUS MARSUPIUM: See GUM KINO.

PTEROCARPUS SANTOLINUS: Same as SANTALUM RUBRUM.

Ptisan: Same as AQUA HORDEUM; later versions were herb infusions (i.e., teas).

PULEGI[UM]: Flowers of the Eurasian pennyroyal, *Mentha*

pulegium, or the American species, *Hedeoma pulegioides*. Aperient, carminative, deobstruent, diaphoretic, antihysteric, and, especially, emmenagogue. [2,15,23,29,30] Occasionally used (unofficially) as an abortifacient today, it can cause severe liver damage. [John B. Sullivan, Jr., Barry H. Rumack, Harold Thomas, Jr., Robert G. Peterson, and Peter Bryson, "Pennyroyal Oil Poisoning and Hepatotoxicity," *Journal of the American Medical Association 242* (1979), 2873-2874]

PULSATILLA NIGRICANS: Meadow anemone or pasqueflower, *Anemone pulsatilla*. Bitter tonic; also applied externally. Side effects include nausea, vomiting, diuresis,and diarrhea, and pain at the site of topical application. [15]

Pulvis: Powder.

PUNICA GRANATUM: See GRANATA MALUS.

Purgative: A strong cathartic.

Putrefacientia: Same as Septa.

Pycnotica: Refrigerant remedies.

PYRETHRUM: Root of Spanish pellitory, *Anacyclus pyrethrum*. A sialagogue that was chewed in order to relieve pains in the head and teeth. [15,29,30] Insecticidal pyrethrum is now obtained from *Chrysanthemum cincerariaefolium*.

Pyriama: Fomentations.

PYRMONT WATER: See PIERMONT WATER.

PYROLA: Leaves of shinleaf, or wintergreen, *Pyrola* spp. Diuretic and digestive; discutient and rubefacient when applied externally. [30]

PYROLIGNEUM, ACIDUM: "Acid of fired wood." Acetic acid (ACIDUM ACETOSUM) made by the destructive distillation of wood. Used to manufacture acetates.

Pyrotica: Escharotics.

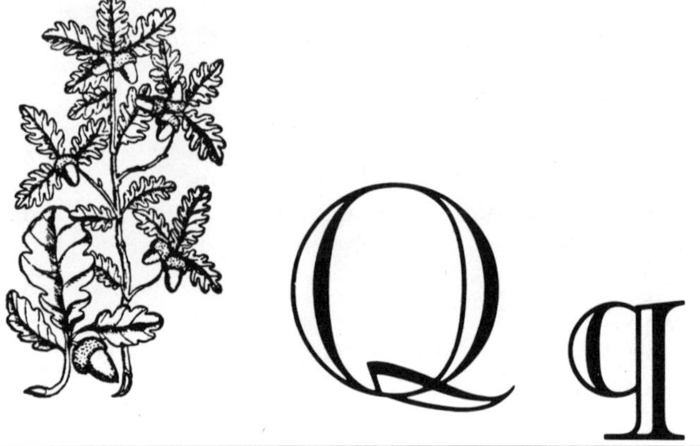

Quercus

QUASSIA [EXCELSA]: Bark of quassy tree, or Surinam quassia, *Quassia amara*, or *Q.* (or *Picrasma*) *excelsa*. Introduced from South America to Europe by British botanist Daniel Solander about 1780. Bitter tonic, antispasmodic, antiemetic, febrifuge, and antiseptic. [2,15,29,30]

QUASSIA SIMAROUBA: Same as SIMAROUBA.

QUEEN-ANNE'S LACE: See DAUCUS SYLVESTRIS.

QUEEN'S DELIGHT (or QUEEN'S-ROOT): See STILLINGIA.

QUERCETANUS'S EXTRACT OF OPIUM: Extract of OPIUM in ACETUM (i.e., vinegar), ascribed to early 17th-century French Paracelsian physician Joseph Duchesne, also known as Quercetanus. Jarcho has perceived that the morphine in the opium would have combined with the acetic acid in the vinegar to produce the first synthesis of heroin, which is diacetylmorphine [40, p. 309].

QUERCETANUS, STOMACHIC POWDER OF: Made of ARUM, CALAMUS, PIMPINELLA, LIXIVA, and CANCRORUM LAPILLI.

QUERCUS ALBA: White oak, *Quercus alba*. An American

oak that can substitute for the European QUERCUS ROBUR. [30]

QUERCUS CERRIS: See GALLA.

QUERCUS [ROBUR]: Bark of the English oak, *Quercus robur*. Strong astringent, tonic, and antiseptic. [2,15,23,29,30] Also see GALLA.

QUERCUS TINCTORIA: Same as QUERCUS ROBUR.

QUICK-GRASS: See GRAMEN.

QUICKLIME: Calcium oxide. Tonic, astringent, and escharotic. [23,29]

QUICKSILVER: Same as HYDRARGYRUS PURIFICATUS.

QUINCE: See CYDONIA MALUS.

QUININE (or QUINIA): See CINCHONA.

QUINQUINA: Same as CINCHONA.

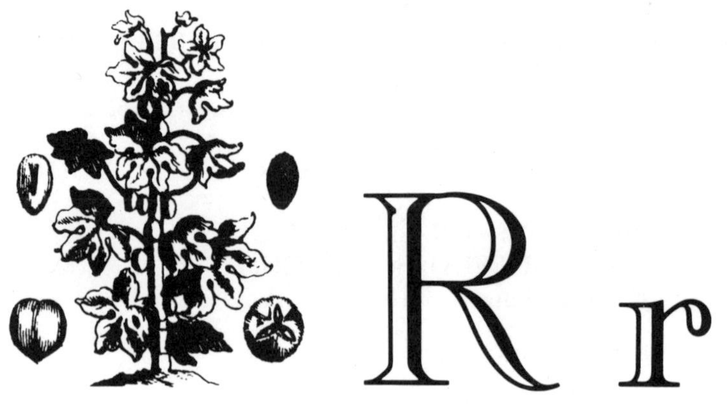

Ricinus

RADCLIFFE'S [PURGING] ELIXIR: Many formulas were derived from the one devised by Dr. John Radcliffe of London about 1700; most contained ALOES, JALAP, GENTIAN, SCAMMONIUM, and SENNA, although one was made with ALOES, CINNAMOMUM, ZEDOARIA, RHEI, COCHINEAL, and RHAMNUS CATHARTICUS.

RAISINS: See UVA PASSA.

RALEIGH, GREAT CORDIAL OF SIR WALTER: Said to have been devised by Raleigh during his imprisonment in the Tower of London in 1603-1616, it was a complex mixture of about 40 plant parts macerated in wine and then distilled. Its formula was later modified as AROMATIC ELECTUARY, def. no. 2. [13]

RALEIGHANA, CONFECTIO: Almost same as def. no. 2 for AROMATIC ELECTUARY, but with 25 ingredients.

Ramich: A tonic and astringent troche.

RANIS, EMPLASTRUM DE: "Frog plaster;" same as EMPLASTRUM VIGONIUM.

RANUNCULUS: Root and stalk of bulbous buttercup, *Ran-*

unculus bulbosus. Used topically as a rubefacient and blister; too poisonous for internal use. [29,30]

RAPHANI COMPOSITUS, SPIRITUS: "Compound spirit of horse radish," made with RAPHANUS RUSTICANUS, CORTEX AURANTIUM, COCHLEARIA HORTENSIS, bruised NUTMEG, and PROOF SPIRIT; sometimes also included ARUM. Antiscorbutic, but abandoned as ineffective by 1790s. [15]

RAPHANUS RUSTICANUS: Root of horse radish, *Armoracia rusticana* or *A. lapathifolia.* Tonic, diuretic, and diaphoretic. [15,23,29] Contains a volatile oil like that found in SINAPI NIGRA.

RASPBERRY: See RUBUS IDAEUS.

RATTLESNAKE ROOT: See SENECA.

RAWSON'S BITTERS: An American "quack remedy" probably made with SANGUINARIA CANADENSIS.

REALGAR: Orange-red arsenic disulfide, As_2S_2.

RED LEAD: Lead tetroxide, Pb_3O_4. Applied externally to cutaneous inflammations. [2,15,23]

RED PRECIPITATE [OF MERCURY]: 1) Same as HYDRARGYRUS NITRATUS RUBER. 2) In the 20th century, mercuric oxide.

RED SULPHURETUM OF QUICKSILVER: Same as HYDRARGYRUS SULPHURATUS RUBER.

Refectiva: Restorative remedies, including tonics.

Refrigerant: An agent that diminishes the force of the circulation and, therefore, reduces body heat, but without decreasing tissue irritability or nervous energy; often also causes diaphoresis or diuresis. Used for inflammations and fevers.

REGENERATED TARTAR: Same as LIXIVA ACETATA.

REGIA, AQUA: Fuming mixture of hydrochloric and nitric acids, it was called "Royal water" because it dissolves gold, the "king of metals."

REGINA, HERBA: See HERBA REGINA.

Relaxantia: Emollient and mildly cathartic remedies that soften the humors and carry them out with the feces.

Repellentia: Astringents that prevent movement of the humors.

REQUIES NICOLAI: "Nicolai's rest," a somnifacient made with OPIUM, HYOSCYAMUS, and MANDRAGORA; invented by Nicolai Myrepsus, a 13th-century Byzantine physician of Nicea.

RESINA ALBA: "White pine resin." Same as TEREBINTHA VENETA.

RESINA FLAVA: "Yellow pine resin." Usually same as TEREBINTHA VULGARIS.

Resolutiva: Resolvents.

Resolvents: Remedies that resolve (i.e., dissolve and disperse) the humors, casting them off through the exhaled air or the circulation.

Restoratives: Tonics.

Restringent: Astringent.

Resumptiva: Pectoral and alimentary remedies that strengthen patients who have been weakened by illness.

RHABARBARUM: Same as RHEI.

RHABARBATATE: Pertaining to RHEI.

RHAMNUS CATHARTICUS: Berries of buckthorn, *Rhamnus catharticus*. Strong cathartic; also said to be tonic, astringent, and antiseptic. Side effects include colic, nausea, and dry mouth. [15,23,29,30]

RHAPONTICUM: Root of monks' rhubarb, *Rheum rhaponticum*. Cathartic, but less potent than RHEI. [15]

RHASIS ALBUM: See ALBUM RHASIS.

RHATANY: See KRAMERIA.

RHEI: Literally, abbreviation of Radix Rhei, root of officinal or Chinese rhubarb, *Rheum officinalis* or *R. palmatum*, but sometimes other species. Mild cathartic, astringent, tonic, stomachic, and antiemetic. Its principal side effect is abdominal pain, caused by excessive stimulation of intestinal activity. Often prepared with added CARDAMOMUM MINUS, ZINGIBER, GLYCERRHIZA, SERPENTINA, and/or SAFFRON, to provide added stomachic and corroborant effects. [1,2,15,23,29] Still used as a cathartic because of its ability to irritate the colon and hasten passage of the stool.

RHEI COMPOSITAE, PILULE: "Compound pill of rhubarb," made with RHEI, ALOES, MYRRH, and OL MENTHA PIPERITA. A tonic cathartic. [23]

RHEUM [PALMATUM or UNDULATUM]: Same as RHEI.

RHEUMATIC WEED: In U.S., same as CHIMAPHILA.

RHODINUM: A mixture of OL ROSARUM and ACETUM.

RHODIUM: See LIGNUM RHODIUM.

RHODODENDRON: *Rhododendron* spp. Its medical use was promoted by Dr. Alexander Bernard Koeplin of Germany in 1779; he called it the Siberian snow rose. Anodyne, narcotic, diaphoretic, and anti-inflammatory, for joint diseases. Side effects included fever, thirst, delirium, "a peculiar creeping like sensation," and vomiting. [15,23] The active poisonous principle, grayanotoxin I (formerly called andromedotoxin or acetylandromedol), was isolated from another genus in 1882, and from rhododendrons in 1887. Because it blocks sodium channels in excitable membranes, its effects include salivation, vomiting, paresthesias (especially around the mouth), skeletal muscle weakness, hypotension, bradycardia, and other cardiac arrhythmias, although death seldom results. [See Kenneth F. Lampe, "Rhododendrons, Mountain Laurel, and Mad Honey," *Journal of the American Medical Association 259* (1988): 2009]

RHOEAS: Same as PAPAVER ERRATICUM.

RHUBARB OF PERU: Same as MECHOACANNA.

RHUS COPALLINUM: Berries of narrow-leaved sumac, *Toxicodendron* (or *Rhus*) *copallina*. Acidic astringent. [23] Non-poisonous. Also see COPAL.

RHUS GLABRUM: Berries of Pennsylvania, or smooth, sumac, *Rhus glabrum*. Acid astringent. [23,29] Non-poisonous.

RHUS RADICANS: Leaves of common poison ivy, *Toxicodendron* (or *Rhus*) *radicans*. Properties like those of RHUS TOXICODENDRON. [23]

RHUS TOXICODENDRON: Leaves of oakleaf poison ivy, *Toxicodendron* (or *Rhus*) *toxicarium*. A potent skin vesicant, although some people are not affected by it. [1,23] Dr. John Alderson of Hull, who first promoted it in his *Essay on the Rhus toxicodendron, or Sumach, with Cases Shewing it's Efficacy in the Cure of Paralytic Affections*, 2nd ed. (Hull: 1794), explicitly avoided discussing the site and mode of this drug's action, but he apparently inferred that it stimulated the nerves in a manner analogous to poison ivy's irritating effect on the skin; perhaps he saw an analogy with blistering agents such as CANTHARIS.

RHUS TYPHINUM: Berries of staghorn sumac, *Toxicodendron* (or *Rhus*) *typhina*. Acidic astringent. [23] Non-poisonous.

RHUS VERNIX: Leaves of poison sumac, *Toxicodendron vernix*. Properties like those of RHUS TOXICODENDRON.

Rhyptica: Detergents.

RIBES NIGRUM: Black currants, *Ribes nigrum*. Used in a syrup for sore throat. [15,23]

RIBES RUBRUM: Red currants, *Ribes rubrum*. Used in a cooling syrup for sore throat. [15,23]

RICE: See ORYZA.

RICINI, OL (or RICINUS [COMMUNIS]): Oil expressed from seeds of castor bean, *Ricinus communis*. Although used since antiquity, it was neglected for two centuries before its reintroduction, from Jamaica, by Dr. Peter Canvane of Bath, England, in 1764. A safe, mild, and demulcent cathartic; sometimes used as a vermifuge. [1,2,15,23,29,30] The active ingredient, ricinoleic acid, was identified by pharmacologist Hans Horst Meyer in 1890; it stimulates fluid secretion and inhibits electrolyte absorption by intestinal mucosal cells, inhibits smooth muscle activity, and possesses antibacterial activity. The seeds also contain ricin, a highly toxic agglutinin that is removed during preparation of the oil. [See Timothy S. Gaginella and Sidney F. Phillips, "Ricinoleic Acid (Castor Oil) Alters Intestinal Surface Structure," *Mayo Clinic Proceedings 51* (1976): 6-12; T. S. Gaginella, A. C. Haddad, V. L. W. Go, and S. F. Phillips, "Cytotoxicity of Ricinoleic Acid (Castor Oil) and Other Intestinal Secretagogues on Isolated Intestinal Epithelial Cells," *Journal of Pharmacology and Experimental Therapeutics 201* (1977): 259-266]

Rob (or Robub): A juice that has been evaporated over heat to the consistency of oil or honey; from Arabic word for curdled milk.

ROBORANS, EMPLASTRUM: "Tonic plaster." Usually, same as EMPLASTRUM THURIS COMPOSITUM; another version contained WHITE LEAD, RESINA ALBA, CERA FLAVA, OL OLIVA, and COLCOTHAR.

Roborantia: Tonics.

ROCHELLE SALT: Same as CREAM OF TARTAR; see SEIGNETTE'S SALT.

ROCHE'S EMBROCATION: Compounded oil of ALNUS, CHAMAEMELUM, CARUM, ROSMARINUS, COCHINEAL, and ALKANET; patented in 1803.

ROCKET: See ERUCA.

ROCK OIL: See PETROLEUM.

ROFFO'S PILL: Correct name for RUFUS'S PILL, although the identity of Roffo is not known.

ROHUN TREE: See SOYMIDA.

ROSA CANINA: Same as CYNOSBATUS.

ROSA DAMASCENA (or PALLIDA): Petals of the damask

rose, *Rosa damascena*. A "cheerful tonic" that does not increase body heat; mild cathartic. [15,23]

ROSAE, AQUA: Rose water, made with ROSA DAMASCENA. Cathartic. [15]

ROSA GALLICA: Petals of French, or common, red rose, *Rosa* spp. Aromatic, astringent, and tonic. [23,29]

ROSARUM, INFUSUM (or TINCTURA): Water extract of dried red rose-buds mixed with dilute VITRIOL. Mild refrigerant and astringent; also used as a gargle. Its effects are attributable to its vitriol content. [15]

ROSATUM PERLATUM: "Pearled rose." Same as DIAMARGARITUM SIMPLEX.

ROSATUM, UNGUENTUM: "Rose ointment." Similar to modern cold cream, which is made of SPERMACETI, CERA ALBA, OL AMYGDALA, AQUA ROSAE, and oil of roses.

ROSE, DOG: See CYNOSBATUS.

ROSEMARY: See ROSMARINUS.

ROSEMARY, MARSH: See STATICE LIMONIUM.

ROSES, CONSERVE OF: Jelly made of ROSA DAMASCENA, VITRIOL, and sugar. A mucolytic gargle; mitigates the side effects of CALOMEL and BLEEDING; a tonic; and an analgesic with mild laxative properties. Its effects are attributable to either its VITRIOL or its sugar content. [1,15] Also see CYNOSBATUS.

ROSEWOOD: See LIGNUM RHODIUM.

ROSMARINUS: Leaves, flowers, or oil, of rosemary, *Rosmarinus officinalis*. Antispasmodic, sedative, cephalic, antihysteric, and emmenagogue. Also used as a liniment. [15,23]

ROSSOLIS: A febrifuge made with TINCTURA CINCHONAE, CORIANDRUM, CANELLA, and sugar.

Rotula: A kind of troche or tablet.

Rubefacient: A medicine that reddens or irritates the skin.

RUBIA [TINCTORUM]: Extract of root of madder, *Rubia tinctorum*. Aperient, detergent, deobstruent, diuretic, and emmenagogue; turns urine and bones red, because it contains the dye alizarin. [1,15,23]

RUBINA ANTIMONII: Probably means "antimony rust." Same as MAGNESIA OPALINA.

RUBRUM, BALSAM: A plaster made with RED LEAD. [2]

RUBUS IDAEUS: Fruit of raspberry, *Rubus idaeus* in Europe, *R. strigosus* in North America. Flavoring; refrigerant, visceral tonic, diuretic, and diaphoretic. [15]

RUBUS NIGER: Fruit of the bramble, or blackberry, *Rubus fruticosus*. Slightly astringent. [15]

RUDII, PILULE: A rapid-acting cathartic remedy made with ALOES and COLOCYNTHIS, it was probably named for Rudiae (or Rudius), a town in southern Italy.

RUE: See RUTA.

RUFUS'S PILL: Compounded of ALOES, MYRRH, and CROCUS (or, in early formulas, ABSINTHUM). Commonly attributed to the second-century Roman physician, Rufus of Ephesus, but see ROFFO'S PILL. Cathartic. [2,23]

RUMEX: Sometimes, but erroneously, used for ACETOSA.

RUMEX ACUTUS: Roots of narrow-leaved dock, *Rumex* spp. Uses like those of RUMEX CRISPUS, q.v. [23]

RUMEX AQUATICUS: Same as HYDROLAPATHUM.

RUMEX BRITTANICA: Same as HYDROLAPATHUM.

RUMEX CRISPUS: Roots of curly-leaved, sour, or yellow dock, *Rumex crispus*. Cathartic; also used in ointments for skin cancer and itch. [23] Contains SAL ACETOSELLAE, q.v.).

RUMEX OBTUSIFOLIUS: Root of broad-leaved, or bitter, dock, *Rumex obtusifolius*. Astringent and laxative. [30]

RUPELLENIS, SAL: "Rochelle salt." Same as CREAM OF TARTAR; see SEIGNETTE'S SALT.

RUSCUS: Rhizomes of butcher's broom, or knee holly, *Ruscus aculeatus*. Deobstruent, diuretic, and diaphoretic. [15]

RUTA [GRAVEOLENS]: Rue, *Ruta graveolens*. Strong tonic, attenuant, detergent, deobstruent, diuretic, diaphoretic, antihysteric, emmenagogue, and antispasmodic; circulation stimulant; irritates the skin and raises blisters if handled too much. [15,23,29]

RYE: See SECALE CORNUTUM.

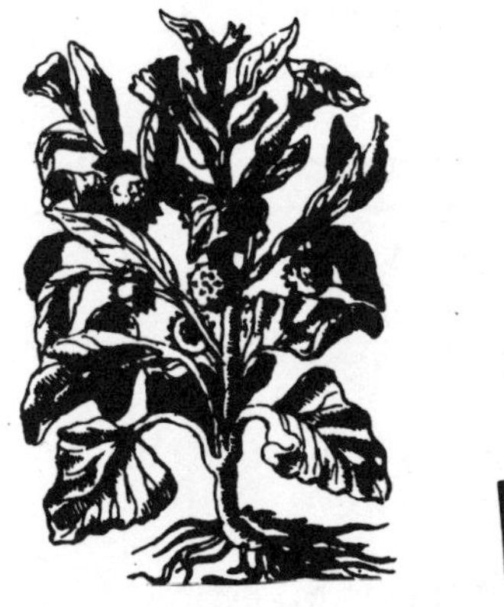

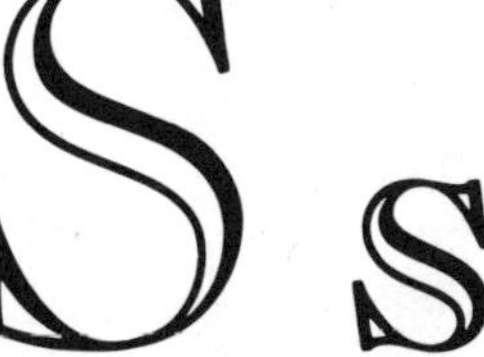

Stramonium

SABADILLA: Seeds and fruit of sabadilla, or cevadilla, *Schoenocaulon officinale*, introduced from tropical America to Europe in 1572, but not promoted as a remedy until the 18th century. Drastic emetic and cathartic; occasionally used as an anthelminthic. [29] Contains veratrine, which K. F. W. Meissner of Halle isolated from sabadilla in 1818; also see VERATRUM entries.

SABBATIA: Rose-pink, bitter bloom, or American centaury, *Sabatia angularis*. Tonic; digestive. [29,30]

SABIN, or SABINA: Leaves of *Juniperus sabina*. Warm, stimulating; aperient, diuretic, diaphoretic, deobstruent, vermifuge, and potent emmenagogue. [15,23,29,30] Also see JUNIPERUS COMMUNIS.

SABINAE COMPOSITA, TINCTURA: "Compound tincture of sabin." Alcohol extract of SABIN, CASTOR, and MYRRH. Used to stimulate menses. [15]

SACCHARUM ALBUM: "White sugar;" same as SACCHARUM PURIFICATUM.

SACCHARUM CANTUM ALBUM et RUBRUM: "White and brown sugar candy."

SACCHARUM NON PURIFICATUM: "Non-purified sugar." Brown sugar.

SACC[HARUM OFFICINARUM]: Sugar, extracted from sugar cane, *Saccharum officinarum*, or, sometimes, molasses. Used for nourishment, as a preservative (in, e.g., conserves, q.v.), or to disguise an unpleasant drug taste. [2,23]

SACCHARUM PENIDIATUM: "Twisted sugar," an anodyne mixture.

SACCHARUM PURIFICATUM: Double refined, or white, sugar.

SACCHARUM SATURNI: "Sugar of lead;" same as CERUSSA ACETATA.

SACRA, TINCTURA: "Sacred tincture," same as VINUM ALOES.

SACRUM, ELIXIR: "Sacred elixir," a tincture of RHEI, Socotrine ALOES, and CARDAMOMUM MINUS. A warming cordial cathartic. [15]

SAFFRON: See CROCUS and CARTHAMUS.

SAGAPENUM: Gum resin of sagapen, probably *Ferula persica* (which resembles ASAFOETIDA). Stimulating aperient, deobstruent, antispasmodic, antihysteric, emmenagogue, and expectorant. [15,29]

SAGE: See SALVIA.

SAGO: Powdery starch obtained from trunks of sago palms, probably *Cycas revoluta*, but perhaps other spp. as well. Used to make a nutritious jelly for convalescents. [15,29]

SALAMANDER BLOOD: See SANG DE SALAMANDRE.

SAL C:C: Usually, an abbreviation for SAL CARBONAS CALCIS, but sometimes for SAL CORNU CERVI.

SALEP, or SALOP: Roots of *Orchis* species; see SATYRION. [2,15]

SALINA, MIXTURA DIAPHORETICA: see JULAP, SALINE.

SALINE: Same as SAL MURIATICUS.

SALINE MIXTURE: Usually same as LIQUOR POTASSAE CITRATIS.

SALINUS AROMATICUS, SPIRITUS: Same as SPIRITUS AMMONIAE AROMATICUS.

SALIX [ALBA]: Bark of white willow, *Salix alba* (or other spp.). Introduced in 1763 as a bitter astringent tonic by Rev. Edward Stone of Oxfordshire, but not widely adopted. Later recommended as a substitute for CINCHONA, but less effective. [15,23,29,30] In 1829 H. Leroux isolated salicin from willow bark; in 1835 salicylic acid was extracted from ULMARIA, and acetylsalicylic acid, aspirin, was synthesized independently by French chemist Charles Frédéric Gerhardt in 1853 and by Felix Hofmann, a Bayer chemist, in 1893. [See H. O. J. Collier, "Aspirin," *Scientific American*, November 1963, pp. 97-108]

SALT OF MANY VIRTUES: Usually same as KALI SULPHURATUM but also see POLYCHRESTUM entries.

SALT OF STEEL: Same as FERRUM VITRIOLATUM.

SALTPETER: Same as SAL NITER.

SALUTIS, ELIXIR: "Elixir of health;" same as TINCTURA SENNAE COMPOSITA; also see DAFFY'S ELIXIR.

SALVIA [OFFICINALIS]: Leaves of sage, *Salvia officinalis*. Warming aromatic, astringent, carminative, tonic appetite stimulant, and nervine. [15,23,29]

SAMBUCUS [NIGRA]: Bark, flowers, and berries of elderberry, *Sambucus niger*. Cathartic, deobstruent, diuretic, and diaphoretic; used as a discutient in poultices. [2,15,23,29]

SAMBUCUS EBULUS: See EBULUS.

SANDALWOOD: See SANTALUM entries.

SANDARACH, GUM: Resin from JUNIPERUS COMMUNIS.

SANDERS: See SANTALUM entries.

SANG DE SALAMANDRE: "Salamander blood," the red residue left after distilling SPIRIT OF NITER. Ancient legends said that salamanders were not harmed by fire.

SANGUINARIA CANADENSIS: Root and seeds of bloodroot, *Sanguinaria canadensis*. Cathartic, tonic, diaphoretic, narcotic, errhine, expectorant, and, because its roots are yellow, a biliary deobstruent; also used for warts. Side effects include heartburn, nausea, vertigo, dim vision, bradycardia, and vomiting. [2,23,29,30]

SANGUIS DRACONIS: "Dragon's blood," the readily flammable gum resin secreted by fruits of the East Indian climbing palms *Daemonorops propinquus* and *D. ruber* (both were originally included in the one species *Calamus draco*) that gives a deep red color in alcohol solution. Astringent and incrassating tonic. Replaced by BRAZIL WOOD and GUM KINO. [See Torald Sollman, "A Sketch of the History of 'Dragon's Blood,'" *Journal of the American Pharmaceutical Association 9* (1920): 141-144.

SANICLE: An herb of genus *Sanicula*, e.g., *S. gregaria*. Astringent.

SANTALUM CITRINUM: Interior wood of yellow sandalwood, or yellow sanders, most often *Santalum album*. Restorative tonic. [15]

SANTALUM RUBRUM: Interior wood of red sanders, *Pterocarpus santalinus*, from India. Astringent tonic, corroborant, and antivenereal; but used chiefly as flavoring and coloring. Often replaced by BRAZIL WOOD. [15]

SANTONICUM: Worm seed, *Artemisia santonicum* and other spp. Anthelminthic. [15,23,29] Santonin, the active principle, was isolated in 1830 by both Kahler, in Düsseldorf, and Augustus Alms, in Mecklenburg–Schwerin; it is effective chiefly against round worms.

SAPA: The residue left after raisins, or hard grapes, are evaporated over fire to the consistency of honey.

SAPIENTIAE, SAL: "Salt of wisdom;" same as SAL ALEMBROTH.

SAPO ALBUS [HISPANUS]: "White [Spanish] soap." Hard soap made with OL OLIVA and LYE; Castilian soap. Administered internally, as a vehicle for resinous drugs, or for its cathartic, antacid, and antilithic properties. [29]

SAPO MOLLIS: Common "soft soap," made with coarse oils, fat, or tallow (but not OL OLIVA), and LYE. More penetrating and acrimonious than SAPO ALBUS; used for external medications. [15]

SAPONACEOUS PILLS: OPIUM or RHEI pills made with SAPO because it promotes absorption of the active ingredients. [2]

SAPONARIA: Root of soapwort, or bruisewort, *Saponaria officinalis*. Aperient, corroborant, and diaphoretic. [15]

SAPO NIGER: "Black soap," like SAPO MOLLIS, but made with LYE and train-oil obtained from whale blubber, seal oil, or fish. [15]

SAPO, VENETIAN: Venetian soap, same as SAPO ALBUS.

SAPPHIRE WATER: Same as AQUA AERUGINIS AMMONIATAE. The copper salt gave it a sapphire color.

SARCOCOLLA: Gum resin from an unknown Arabian or Persian plant. Astringent and detergent vulnerary. [15]

Sarcotica: Remedies that promote wound healing; vulneraries.

SARSAPARILLA: Usually, the powdered root of *Smilax aristolochiaefolia* or *S. ornata* introduced to Spain from South

America in 1530; introduced to France as an antirheumatic in 1556 and as an antivenereal in 1563. However, sometimes refers to North American species, especially the bristly sarsaparilla, *Aralia hispida*, or wild or false sarsaparilla, *A. nudicaulis*. Used chiefly as flavoring or for venereal disease in the 18th century, and as a mild demulcent all-purpose tonic and diaphoretic by the mid-19th century. [1,7,23,29,30]

SARSAPARILLAE COMPOSITUM, DECOCTUM: Made with SARSAPARILLA, SASSAFRAS, GUAIAC, GLYCERRHIZA, and MEZEREUM. Tonic diet drink. [15]

SASSAFRAS: Wood, root, and bark of *Sassafras albidum*. Introduced from North America by Spanish, French, and English explorers in the late 16th century. Aperient, tonic, blood purifier, diuretic, diaphoretic, antirheumatic, and antisyphilitic. [2,23,29,30]

SATUREIA: Summer savory, *Satureia hortensis*. Aromatic. [15]

SATURN: Lead; see PLUMBUM and definitions immediately below.

SATURN, EXTRACT OF: Same as CERUSSA ACETATA; also see GOULARD'S EXTRACT OF SATURN.

SATURNINE ANODYNE PILLS: "Lead analgesic pills." Made of CERUSSA ACETATA, IPECAC, and OPIUM. [2]

SATURNINE OINTMENT: Made with 20 parts SIMPLE OINTMENT and one part CERUSSA ACETATA. A plaster with refrigerant properties. [2]

SATURNI, SACCHARUM: "Sugar of lead." Same as CERUSSA ACETATA.

SATYRION: Root of *Orchis mascula* (because its flowers resemble the scrotum, it was associated with the priapic power of satyrs), or perhaps other spp. (e.g., the downy rattlesnake plantain, *Goodyera pubescens*, a small American orchid). Analeptic, aphrodisiac, and other tonic actions. [15] Nutritive; antidiarrheal demulcent. [23]

SAUCE-ALONE: See ALLIARIA.

SAUERKRAUT: See BRASSICA.

SAUNDERS: Same as SANDERS; see SANTALUM entries.

SAVINE: Same as SABIN.

SAVORY, SUMMER: See SATUREIA.

SAXIFRAGE, BURNET: See PIMPINELLA.

SCAMMONII COMPOSITUS, PULVIS: "Compound powder of scammony." 1) In London, made with SCAMMONIUM, JALAP, and ZINGIBER. Cathartic. 2) In Edinburgh, made with SCAMMONIUM and CREAM OF TARTAR. Cathartic, but its warming property is ameliorated by the cream of tartar. [15]

SCAMMONII, ELECTUARIUM: "Electuary of scammony." Made with SCAMMONIUM, CARYOPHYLLUS AROMATICUS, ZINGIBER, CARUM, and SYRUPUS ROSARUM. Warm, brisk cathartic. [15]

SCAMMONIUM: Gum resin of scammony, or Syrian bindweed, *Convolvulus scammonia*. Strong cathartic, sometimes hazardous. [1,2,15,23,29] Its active cathartic principle is also found in JALAP.

SCARIFICATION: See BLEEDING.

Scelotyrbica: Remedies for scorbutic limbs.

SCILLA [MARITIMA]: Bulb of squill, or sea onion, *Urginea* (or *Scilla*) *maritima*. Diuretic, expectorant, and diaphoretic; emetic and cathartic at high doses. [15,23,29; also see "Symposium on Squill," *Bulletin of the New York Academy of Medicine 50* (1974): 682-750] Contains DIGITALIS-like glycosides called scillarens that are not therapeutically dependable.

SCILLAE, or SCILLITICAE, PILULE: "Squill pill," usually made with SCILLA, GUM AMMONIAC, GLYCERRIHIZA, CARDAMOMUM MINUS, and simple syrup. Used chiefly as a strong diuretic, but occasionally as a diaphoretic or sialagogue, especially before the introduction of DIGITALIS in 1785; cathartic in high doses. [1,2,15,23,30]

Sclerontica: Remedies that harden the flesh.

SCOLOPENDRIUM: Leaves of harts-tongue fern, *Scolopendrium vulgare*. Deobstruent and visceral tonic. [15]

SCOPARIUS: Fresh tops of broom, *Cytisus scoparius*. Diuretic and cathartic; emetic in large doses. [29]

SCORDIUM: Water, or garlic, germander, *Teucrium scordium*. Deobstruent, diuretic, and diaphoretic. [15]

SCOTS PILLS: See ANDERSON'S SCOTS PILLS.

SCROPHULARIA NODOSA: Leaves of figwort, *Scrophularia* spp. (perhaps *S. marilandica*). Anodyne, astringent, diuretic, tonic, diaphoretic, discutient, and anthelminthic; especially useful in treating scrofula. [29]

Scruple (or Scrupulus): See Measurement.

SCULLCAP: See SCUTELLARIA LATERIFOLIA.

SCURVYGRASS: See COCHLEARIA HORTENSIS.

SCURVYGRASS, SCOTS: See BRASSICA MARINA.
SCURVYGRASS, SEA: See COCHLEARIA MARINA.
SCUTELLARIA LATERIFOLIA: Blue scullcap, hooded willow herb, or mad-dog skull cap, *Scutellaria laterifolia.* Remedy for rabies. [23]

Scutum: 1) An alcohol-based plaster applied over the heart or stomach to strengthen it. 2) Same as an Ecusson.

SEA COLEWORT: See BRASSICA MARINA.
SEA HOLLY: See ERYNGIUM.
SEA LAVENDER: See STATICE LIMONIUM.
SEA ONION: See SCILLA.
SEBESTENA: Sebestens, the mucilaginous sweet plum-like fruits of *Cordia myxa*. Used for hoarseness and cough. [15]

SEBUM: "Fat," suet from mutton, beef, ram, or billy-goat; also see AXUNGUENTUM PORCINUM.

SEBUM CASTRATI: "Weak [or thin] fat." Suet from a ram.

SECALE CORNUTUM: "Spurred rye," or ergot, is the sclerotium, or dormant stage, of a fungus, *Claviceps purpurea*, that grows on rye, *Secale cereale.* First recommended for obstetrical use by botanist Adam Lonicer of Frankfurt in 1582, and reintroduced in 1787. Although in 1807 Dr. John Stearns of New York recommended it to hasten birth, and Dr. David Hosack of New York recommended it for the control of postpartum hemorrhage in 1824, its use remained controversial. Side effects include vomiting, headache, mydriasis, delirium, and stupor, as well as fetal death. [23,29,30] The several ergot alkaloids, especially ergotamine (extracted in 1864 and isolated by A. Stoll in 1920), have complex effects; their major uses today are as oxytocics and for migraine. [See Frank J. Bove, *The Story of Ergot* (Basel: S. Karger, 1970)]

Sedative: A drug that diminishes irritability and sensibility; also see Narcotics.

SEDATIVUS HOMBERGII, SAL: See HOMBERG'S NARCOTIC SALT.

SEDATUM, SAL: "Sedative salt." Made by volatilizing SAL MURIATICUS and VITRIOL with BORACIS.

SEDUM ACRE: Fresh stone-crop, *Sedum acre*. Emetic, cathartic, and diuretic. [15]

SEIDLITZ POWDERS: Named, by mistake, for SEIDLITZ SALT, this product was sold as two powders, one of tartaric acid (15 grains), the other a mixture of CREAM OF TARTAR (2 drachms) and sodium bicarbonate (2 scruples), to be dissolved in a half-pint of water before drinking. Patented by apothecary Thomas Field Savory of London in 1815. Cathartic.

SEIDLITZ SALT: Same as MAGNESIA VITRIOLATA. The medicinal value of a mineral spring at Seidlitz, in Bohemia, was discovered by Dr. Friedrich Hoffmann of Halle in 1724; its waters also contained VITRIOLATED SODA.

SEIGNETTE'S SALT: Same as CREAM OF TARTAR, independently discovered by apothecary Pierre Seignette of LaRochelle, France, in 1662. [13]

SELF-HEAL: See PRUNELLA.

SELTZER WATER: A SODA WATER originally found at Selters, near Wiesbaden, Germany, it contained SAL MURIATICUS, CARBONAS SODAE, and SUPER-CARBONATIS SODAE; a synthetic carbonated version was being manufactured in the U.S. by about 1809. Diuretic, febrifuge, antacid, and expectorant; prescribed for dyspepsia, catarrh, and urinary tract stones. [23] The therapeutic idea behind the medical use of Seltzer water survives in products such as "Alka-Seltzer," although it is composed of SUPER-CARBONATIS SODAE, ACIDUM CITRICUM, and SUPER–CARBONATIS POTASSAE.

SENECA (or SENEGA or SENEKA): Seneca snakeroot, or rattlesnake root, *Polygala senega*. Introduced by Dr. John Tennent of Virginia in the 1730s. Tonic, expectorant, anti-inflammatory, diuretic, diaphoretic, sialagogue, and cathartic; emetic in high dose. [15,23,29,30]

SENECA OIL: American term for PETROLEUM.

SENECIO: See GROUNDSEL.

SENNA: Leaves of *Cassia acutifolia*, *C. angustifolia*, or other spp. Cathartic; diuretic. Side effects include severe abdominal pain and a bad taste in the mouth. [1,2,15,23,29,30] Still used as a cathartic by virtue of its ability to irritate the colon.

SENNA, AMERICAN: Wild senna, *Cassia marilandica*; see CASSIA FISTULA.

SENNAE COMPOSITA, TINCTURA: "Compound tincture of senna." Alcohol extract of SENNA, JALAP, and CORIANDRUM. Carminative and cathartic. [2,15]

SENNAE, CONFECTIO: Same as BENEDICTA LAXATIVA.

SENNAE SIMPLEX, INFUSUM: "Simple infusion of senna," made with SENNA and ZINGIBER.

SENNAE TARTARISATUM, INFUSUM: "Tartarized infusion of senna." Made with SENNA, CORIANDRUM, and CREAM OF TARTAR. The latter makes the taste tolerable and promotes the drug's cathartic action. [15]

SENTINELLE, POWDER OF: Same as MAGNESIA ALBA.

Seplasaria: Simple aromatic unguents.

Septa: External remedies that corrode the flesh and promote suppuration.

SEPTFOIL: See TORMENTILLA.

SERPENTARIA [VIRGINIANA]: Root of Virginia snakeroot, *Aristolochia serpentaria*. Introduced from Virginia to England by 1632. Tonic, diuretic, diaphoretic, antispasmodic, anodyne, and alexipharmic; increases pulse; potentiates CINCHONA. Sometimes used in enemas. Side effects include colic and vomiting. [1,2,15,23,29,30]

SERPENTINA: Same as SERPENTARIA.

SERPYLLUM: Flowers of mother-of-thyme, *Thymus serpyllum*. Properties like those of THYMUS, but weaker. [15]

SESAMUM ORIENTALE: Oil from sesame seeds, or benne, from *Sesamum indicum*. Gentle mucilaginous laxative. [23,29]

SETON: A thread or other fibrous material passed through subcutaneous tissue to facilitate the release of serum or pus, for the same therapeutic reasons that blisters are raised with CANTHARIS. [1]

SEVUM [OVILLUM]: Same as OVIS.

SEVUM CETI: Same as SPERMACETI.

SHELLAC: See LACCA.

SHEPHERD'S PURSE: See BURSA PASTORIS.

Sialagogue: A drug that increases salivary discharge. No therapeutic usefulness was attributed to the enhanced salivation *per se*, although the saliva was understood to be a suitable exit portal for disturbed humors or contagious elements (e.g., the "virus" of syphilis when treated with HYDRARGYRUS).

SIBERIAN SNOW ROSE: See RHODODENDRON.

SILESIAN EARTH: A brownish BOLUS that does not react with acids.

SILPHIUM: In the ancient world, probably a cathartic extract of *Ferula tingitana* or other related species, but perhaps the deadly carrot, *Thapsia garganica*; after about 100 A.D., ASAFOETIDA was meant. The North American genus of rosin weeds, *Silphium*, seems not to have been used in medicine. [See Chalmers L. Gemmill, "Silphium," *Bulletin of the History of Medicine 40* (1966): 295-313]

SIMAROUBA: Bark of mountain damson, *Simarouba amara* or *S. officinalis*. Introduced from Guyana to France in 1713. Bitter tonic, astringent, cathartic, and emetic. [15,23,29,30]

Simple Syrup: Usually made by dissolving 15 parts of SACCHARUM PURIFICATUM in eight parts water over heat.

SIMPLEX, EMPLASTRUM: Same as EMPLASTRUM CERAE COMPOSITUM.

SINAPI [ALBA or NIGRA]: White or black mustard seed, respectively, from *Brassica alba* and *B. nigra*. Appetite stimulant, digestive, diuretic, diaphoretic, emetic, laxative, and antiscorbutic. Often used in SINAPISMS as a rubefacient or mild blistering agent. [15,23,29,30] The blistering alkaloids in the two species are chemically similar, and are still used to make mustard plasters.

SINAPISM: A cataplasm made with SINAPI.

SINGLETON'S GOLDEN EYE OINTMENT: A proprietary verison of CITRINE OINTMENT.

SIROEUM: Same as SAPA.

SIUM: Water parsnip, *Sium latifolium* or *S. nodiflorum*. Diuretic, emmenagogue, and lithontriptic. [15]

SKUNK CABBAGE: See ARUM AMERICANUM.

SLIPPERY ELM: See ULMUS RUBRA.

SLOE: See PRUNUS SYLVESTRIS.

SMALLAGE: See APIUM.

SMALL BEER: Weak beer containing about 1.2% alcohol. Weak tonic. Also see PORTER.

SMARTWEED: See PERSICARIA.

Smecticum: A remedy for cleaning the skin.

Smegma: Same as Smecticum.

SMELLON'S EYE-SALVE: A proprietary copper-based ointment much like UNGUENTUM AERUGINIS.

SMILAX CHINA: See CHINA.

SMILAX SARSAPARILLA: Same as SARSAPARILLA.

SNAKEROOT: 1) Same as SERPENTARIA. 2) In U.S., sometimes meant white snakeroot, *Eupatorium rugosum*. Astringent and diuretic. Contains tremetol, which was responsible for the early 19th-century epidemics of "milksickness" characterized by vomiting, weakness, constipation, tremors, delirium, and high mortality. 3) Also see CIMIFUGA and SENECA.

SNAKEWEED: See BISTORTA.

SNAKEWOOD: Wood or roots of *Strychnos colubrina*. Narcotic and tonic bitter, like NUX VOMICA. [15]

SNEEZEWORT: See PTARMICA.

SNUFF: Finely pulverized NICOTIANA. An errhine drawn into the nostrils by inhalation, to facilitate the release of phlegm. [1]

SOAP: See SAPO entries.

SOAPWORT: See SAPONARIA.

SOCOT[O]RINE ALOES: See ALOES.

SODA: Usually, same as BARILLA.

SODA ASH: Same as CARBONAS SODAE.

SODAE ACETAS: Sodium acetate. Diuretic, but used chiefly in the manufacture of ACETUM ACETOSUM.

SODAE BORAS: Same as BORAX.

SODAE CARBONAS: Same as CARBONAS SODAE.

SODAE CARBONAS IMPURA (or VENALE): Same as BARILLA.

SODAE SULPHAS: Same as VITRIOLATED SODA.

SODA PHOSPHORATA: Sodium phosphate. Introduced about 1785 by Dr. Pearson of London. Pleasant cooling cathartic for inflammatory diseases. [1,15,23,30]

SODA TARTARISATA: Same as CREAM OF TARTAR.

SODA VITRIOLATA: Same as VITRIOLATED SODA.

SODA WATER: Water impregnated with FIXED AIR. In 1772, Rev. Joseph Priestley, then at Leeds, described the necessary processes, and it was being manufactured in the U.S. from about 1809. Diaphoretic, diuretic, and a digestive antacid for stomach complaints and urinary tract stones. [23,29]

SODII CHLORIDUM: Same as SAL MURIATICUS.

SOLANUM DULCAMARA: Same as DULCAMARA.

SOLANUM LETHALE: Same as BELLADONNA.

SOLDANELLA: See BRASSICA MARINA.

SOLIDAGO: In U.S., sweet-smelling golden rod, *Solidago odora*. Stimulant, carminative, and diuretic. [30] Also see VIRGA AUREA.

SOLID PANACEA: See PANACEA, SOLID.

SOLOMON'S CORDIAL BALM OF GILEAD: An expensive proprietary panacea (said to be especially effective in men suffering from onanism) of unknown composition devised about 1788 by Samuel Solomon of Leeds, England. [William H. Helfand, "Samuel Solomon and the Cordial Balm of Gilead," *Pharmacy in History 31* (1989): 151-159]

SOLOMON'S SEAL: See CONVALLARIA.

SOLUBLE TARTAR: Same as SAL TARTARI.

Solutiva: Cathartics.

Somnifacient: A soporific drug.

Somnifera: Soporific drugs.

SOPHORA TINCTORIA: Wild indigo, or indigo weed, *Baptisia tinctoria.* Emetic, cathartic, and antiseptic. [23] Produces effects like those of CICUTA.

Soporific: A drug that induces sleep, usually a narcotic.

SORREL: See ACETOSA and LUJULA.

SORREL, ACID OF: Oxalic acid; see SAL ACETOSELLAE, LUJULA, RUMEX ACUTUS, and RUMEX CRISPUS.

SOUR WHEY: Lactic acid.

SOUTHERNWOOD: See ABROTANUM.

SOWBREAD: See ARTHANITA.

SOYMIDA: Powdered bark of the rohun tree, *Soymida febrifuga* (but sometimes a mahogany, *Swietenia* spp.), introduced from India to British medicine in the 1790s. Tried—unsuccessfully—as an astringent and gentle tonic, and to reduce irritability, and, because of its tonic property, as a substitute for CINCHONA. Its principal side effect is vertigo. [1; also see Edward John Waring, *Pharmacopoeia of India* (London: India Office, 1868), pp. 55, 444]

SPA WATERS: For the contents of several 19th-century American and European naturally-occurring mineral waters, see ref. 29, pp. 112-115. Also see BALLSTON WATER, PIERMONT WATER, and STAFFORD SPRING WATER.

Sparadrapum: A suppurative plaster in which pieces of linen are soaked while it is still warm, just before applying it to the patient.

SPEARMINT: See MENTHA SATIVA.

Specific: "An antidote, a medicine which cures a [specific] disease by means which physicians do not pretend to explain." [11] Thus, an 18th-century "specific" was not a drug that was selectively effective for a given ailment, but a drug whose efficacy could not be explained by contemporary physiological concepts.

SPECIFICUM PURGANS: "Specific purgative." Same as KALI SULPHURATUM.

SPEEDIMAN'S PILLS: An early 19th-century proprietary cathartic made with ALOES, MYRRH, RHEI, and CHAMAEMELUM.

SPEEDWELL: See BECCABUNGA.

SPERMACETI: Literally, "whale sperm," but really oil from the head of the sperm whale, *Physeter catodon*; relaxing demulcent and emollient used in many lotions, etc., and for catarrh and gonorrhea (i.e., spermatorrhea). [2,6,15,23,29] Its chief ingredient is cetyl palmitate.

SPHONDYLIUM: See HERACLEUM SPHONDYLIUM.

SPIGELIA [MARILANDICA]: Root of Indian pink, or Carolina pinkroot, *Spigelia marilandica*. Introduced to Europe by Drs. John Lining and Alexander Garden of Charleston, S.C., in 1754–1756. Anthelminthic; the convulsions that sometimes follow low doses are minimized by the cathartic or emetic effects of large doses. [15,23,29,30]

SPIGNEL: See MEUM.

SPIKENARD: See NARDUS INDICA.

SPINA CERVINA: Same as RHAMNUS CATHARTICUS.

SPIRAEA TOMENTOSA (or TRIFOLIATA): Root of hardhack, steeplebush, or Indian physic, *Spiraea tomentosa*. Astringent, emetic, and tonic. [23,29,30] Also see ULMARIA.

Spiritus [Distillati or Stillatiti]: Distilled spirits, obtained by distilling plant materials containing alcohol-soluble essential oils in PROOF SPIRIT or other alcohol. Usually volatilize readily.

SPISSATUS, SUCCUS: "Thick juice." Its chief ingredient was SAMBUCUS.

Splanchnica (or Splenetica, or Splenica): Appetite stimulants and remedies for disorders of the spleen.

Spodium: A fine powder obtained by calcination (i.e., oxidation).

SPONDIUM: Burned ivory. Tonic and antacid.

SPONGIA [OFFICINALIS]: Sponge, the absorbent connective tissue structure of invertebrates of the phylum Porifera. Used to clean and cover wounds. [15,29]

SPURGE, FLOWERING: See EUPHORBIA COROLLATA.

SPURGE LAUREL: See MEZEREUM.

SQUILLS: See SCILLAE.

SQUILLS, OXYMEL OF: Drink made of a vinegar extract of SQUILLS and honey. Aperient and expectorant; emetic in large doses. [2,15]

SQUIRE'S GRAND ELIXIR: A proprietary remedy made with OPIUM.

SQUIRTING CUCUMBER: See CUCUMIS AGRESTIS.

ss.: Abbreviation for half of a given weight or volume.

STAFFORD SPRING WATER: From Stafford Spring, Conn. Contained FERRUM salts, FIXED AIR, hydrogen sulfide, and salts of magnesium and aluminum. Tonic. [23, p. 571]

Staltica: Remedies that suppress raised flesh around wounds.

STANNI AMALGAMA: "Amalgam of tin." Powdered mixture of STANNUM and HYDRARGYRUS PURIFICATUS. Anthelminthic. [15]

STANNI, PULVIS: Powdered STANNUM. Anthelminthic. [15,29,30]

STANNUM: Elemental tin. Antihysteric and anthelminthic. [15,23]

STAPHISAGRIA: Seed of stavesacre, *Delphinium staphisagria*. Violent cathartic. Because of its strong emetic effect, used chiefly only for skin eruptions and infestations (e.g., lice). [15,29]

STARKEY'S PILL: An opiate with the same ingredients as in MATTHEW'S PILL, it was devised by 17th-century London physician George Starkey.

STATICE [LIMONIUM]: Root of sea lavender, or marsh rosemary, *Limonium nashii*. Astringent, antiseptic, and expectorant; administered internally and externally. [23,29]

STAVESACRE: See STAPHISAGRIA.

STECHAS: Flowers of stechados, Arabian stechas, or French lavender, *Lavandula stoechas*. Aromatic. [15]

STEEL: Usually synonymous with FERRUM.

STEER'S CELEBRATED (or CHEMICAL) OPODELDOC: Advertised in London in 1780 by Dr. Steer, who added ammonia to the soap liniment version used in Edinburgh. Promoted for about 40 years more as a panacea liniment, but apparently not patented. [14] See OPODELDOC for earlier versions.

Stegnotica: Incrassating drugs.

STEGNOTICUS, PULVIS: "Thickening powder." Same as AETHIOPS VEGETABILIS.

Stephaniaea: Remedies applied over the cranial sutures to stimulate transpiration and to strengthen the neck.

STEPHEN'S [MRS.] CURE FOR STONE: An invention of Mrs. Johanna Stephens, in the 1730s. By a 1739 Act of Parliament, she was paid £5,000 for the formula, which included burned egg shells, whole snails, soap, honey, BARDANA, CHAMAEMELUM, DAUCUS SYVESTRIS, FOENICULUM DULCIS, and PETROSELINUM. [13]

Sternutatory: A snuff used as an errhine.

STERNUTATORY POWDER: "Sneezing powder." Same as PULVIS ASARI COMPOSITUS.

STIBIUM: Same as ANTIMONIUM.

Stictica: Astringent remedies for external use.

ST. IGNATIUS'S BEANS: Seeds of *Strychnos ignatii*. Introduced to Europe by about 1698 by Father Camellus, a Jesuit missionary from Manila, who named it for St. Ignatius Loyola, founder of his order. Narcotic bitter with properties like those of NUX VOMICA. [15,29] Both contain strychnine.

STILLINGIA: Root of queen's-root, or queen's delight, *Stillingia sylvatica*. Introduced by Dr. Thomas Young Simons in 1828, it became a staple ingredient of 19th-century patent medicines. Diaphoretic, alterative, and tonic in small doses; emetic and cathartic in large doses. [7, 29]

Stimulants: Usually, drugs that "raise the actions" of the heart and arteries, as detected by an increased pulse rate, or by reddening of the skin. The therapeutic efficacy of many stimulants was manifested by their evacuant effects, such as diuresis (indicating that the renal arteries had been stimulated) and diaphoresis (indicating that cutaneous vessels had been stimulated). Also see Narcotics and Tonics.

STINKING ORACH: See ATRIPLEX FOETIDA.

ST. JOHN'S WORT: See HYPERICUM.

STOECHAS: Same as STECHAS.

Stomachic: A medicine that warms and strengthens the stomach.

STOMACHICOS, TINCTURA AD: Same as VINUM AMARUM.

STOMACHICUM, ELIXIR: See STOUGHTON'S BITTERS.

STOMACHICUM POTERII: "Stomachic of Poterius." Same as DIAPHORETICUM SOLARE, with GUM TRAGACANTH added; see ANTIHECTICUM POTERII.

Stomatica: Pleasant tasting Detergents.

STONE-CROP: See SEDUM ACRE.

STORAX: See STYRAX CALAMITA.

STOUGHTON'S BITTERS, ELIXIR, or TINCTURE: A mixture of 22 ingredients made by Richard Stoughton of Southwark for 20 years before he patented it in 1712 as "Stoughton's Elixir Magnum Stomachii, or the Great Cordial Elixir, otherwise called the Stomatick Tincture or Bitter Drops;" that is, it was promoted as a tonic panacea for any ailment related to the stomach. Became official in 1762, as Elixir Stomachicum, and later as TINCTURA GENTIANAE COMPOSITUM. [14]

STRAMONIUM: Leaves, roots, and seeds of thornapple, or jimson (Jamestown) weed, *Datura stramonium*. Indigenous to the Old World, it was introduced to medicine as an antiepileptic (although other species of *Datura* had long been known as poisons) by Dr. Anton Störck of Vienna in 1762. Potent narcotic, tonic, diuretic, anodyne, antispasmodic, and antitussive. Its side effects include, as the dose increases, vertigo, headache, dim vision (its dose can be adjusted by the degree of mydriasis produced), confused thought (including delirium and feeling of intoxication), a feeling of suffocation, sleepiness, relaxation of the bowels, diuresis, and diaphoresis, all of which persist for several hours. In larger doses, it produces heart pain, excessive thirst, nausea and vomiting, a sense of strangulation, anxiety, partial or complete blindness, intense delirium ("sometimes of a furious, sometimes of a whimsical character"), tremors, palsy, convulsions, and, sometimes, death. Used chiefly in disorders of the nervous system, including painful syndromes; applied in ointments or poultices to cutaneous inflammations and hemorrhoids, and to the eye to dilate the pupil in preparation for cataract extraction. The berries contain the highest concentration of the active principle, but the leaves are also smoked, especially for treating asthma. [15,23,29,30] Now known to contain antimuscarinic alkaloids, chiefly hyoscyamine, which was isolated from the plant about 1833 by Philipp Lorenz Geiger and Germain Henri Hess, of Heidelberg.

STRASBOURG TURPENTINE: Same as TEREBINTHA ARGENTORATENSIS.

STRAWBERRIES: See FRAGA.

STRENGTHENING PLASTER: Composed of RED LEAD, RESINA FLAVA, CERA FLAVA, and OL OLIVA. Used to strengthen leg muscles. [2]

STRYCHNOS COLUBRINA: See SNAKEWOOD.

STRYCHNOS IGNATII: See ST. IGNATIUS' BEANS.

STRYCHNOS NUX-VOMICA: See NUX VOMICA.

Stupefacientia: Soporifics.

STYGIA, AQUA: "Stygian water," so-called because the water of the mythical River Styx was said to have been as corrosive as AQUA REGIA, q.v.

Stymmata: Aromatic dry materials in oils.

Styptic: A potent astringent.

STYPTICA, AQUA: "Styptic water;" same as AQUA CUPRI VITRIOLATI COMPOSITA.

STYPTICUS [HELVETII], PULVIS: "Styptic powder of Helvetius," made of ALUM and GUM KINO; SANGUIS DRACONIS was included in the earliest formulations. Attributed to 17th-century French physician Adrien Helvetius. Also see PULVIS ALUMINIS COMPOSITUS. Used especially to control uterine hemorrhage and bleeding wounds. [15,23]

STYRACE, PILULE E: "Styrax pill," made with OPIUM (6%), STYRAX CALAMITA, and GLYCERRHIZA. Used chiefly for the effects of OPIUM. [15]

STYRAX BENZOIN: See BENZOIN.

STYRAX CALAMITA: Storax, resin of *Liquidambar orientalis* or perhaps *Styrax officinalis*. Stimulating expectorant. [15,23,29]

SUB-ACETAS (or SUB-ACETIS) CUPRI: Same as VERDEGRIS.

SUB-BORAS SODAE: Same as BORAX.

SUB-CARBONAS AMMONIAE: Same as AMMONIA PRAEPARATA.

SUB-CARBONAS FERRI: Ferric carbonate.

SUB-CARBONAS SODAE: Same as CARBONAS SODAE.

SUB-MURIAS HYDRARGYRI [PRAECIPITATUS]: Same as CALOMEL.

SUB-NITRAS BISMUTHI: Bismuth nitrate. Digestive; antiemetic; tonic, and antispasmodic. [30]

SUB-SULPHAS HYDRARGYRI FLAVUS: Same as HYDRARGYRUS VITRIOLATUS.

SUCCINI, OL: Oil of amber, the fossilized resin of an extinct pine, *Pinites succinifera*. Tonic, antispasmodic, antirheumatic, and antihysteric, but its efficacy is doubtful; also applied topically as a friction, for treating paralysis. [1,23]

SUCCINUM: Amber or its distillation products, OL SUCCINI and SAL SUCCINUM.

SUCCINUM, SAL: Salt of amber, succinic acid. Observed by German mineralogist Georgius Agricola (Georg Bauer) in 1546, and described by Paracelsian chemist Dr. Oswald Croll of Anhalt in 1609. Cathartic, diuretic, and antihysteric. [2,15,23]

SUCCORY: See CICHOREUM.

Succus: A juice expressed from a plant or its fruits.

Sudorific: A strong diaphoretic.

Suffitus (or Suffimenta, or Suffumigia): Aromatic drugs to be burned in the sickroom.

SUGAR: See SACCHARUM entries.

SUGAR OF LEAD: Same as CERUSSA ACETATA.

SULPHAS BARYTAE: Same as BARYTAS.

SULPHAS CUPRI: Same as BLUE VITRIOL.

SULPHAS FERRI [EXSICCATUS]: Same as FERRUM VITRIOLATUM [EXSICCATUM].

SULPHAS MAGNESIAE: Same as MAGNESIA VITRIOLATA.

SULPHAS POTASSAE: Same as KALI SULPHURATUM.

SULPHAS POTASSAE CUM SULPHURE: Same as KALI SULPHURATUM.

SULPHAS SODAE: Same as VITRIOLATED SODA.

SULPHAS ZINCI: Same as ZINCUM VITRIOLATUM.

SULPHATIS CUPRI COMPOSITA, SOLUTIO: Same as AQUA CUPRI VITRIOLATI COMPOSITA.

SULPHUR: Usually means sublimated sulfur, "flowers of sulfur". Cooling cathartic, diaphoretic, and resolvent; antagonizes the side effects of mercury and antimony; also applied to skin disease. [1,23,30] Also see entries beginning with VITRIOL.

SULPHURATUM, OLEUM: "Sulphurated oil," SULPHUR boiled in OL OLIVA. Used internally as a pectoral, although hazardous; usually applied to running sores. [15]

SULPHUR AURATUM ANTIMONII: Same as SULPHUR ANTIMONII PRAECIPITATUM.

SULPHUR, BALSAM OF: Same as OLEUM SULPHURATUM.

SULPHUR, BALSAMUM CRASSUM: Same as OLEUM SULPHURATUM.

SULPHURETUM ANTIMONII: Same as ANTIMONIUM CRUDUM.

SULPHURETUM ANTIMONII PRAECIPITATUM: A variable mixture of ANTIMONIUM and VITRIOL ANTIMONIUM; actually, red antimony sulfide, Sb_2S_5. Emetic. [15]

SULPHURETUM HYDRARGYRUS NIGRUM: Same as HYDRARGYRUS SULPHURATUS NIGER.

SULPHURETUM HYDRARGYRUS RUBRUM: Same as HYDRARGYRUS SULPHURATUS RUBER.

SULPHURETUM POTASSAE: Same as KALI SULPHURATUM.

SULPHUR, FLOWERS OF: Same as SULPHUR.

SULPHURIC ETHER (or AETHER): Same as AETHER VITRIOLICUS.

SULPHURICUM, ACIDUM: Same as OL VITRIOL.

SULPHURICUM AROMATICUM, ACIDUM: Same as ACIDUM VITRIOLI AROMATICUM.

SULPHURICUS CUM ALCOHOLE, AETHER: AETHER VITRIOLICUS diluted with alcohol, but no more effective than the undiluted compound. [23]

SULPHUR LOTUM [SUBLIMATUM]: "Washed SULPHUR."

SUPER-CARBONATIS FERRI, AQUA: Solution of ferrous carbonate. Tonic. [23]

SUPER–CARBONATIS POTASSAE: Potassium bicarbonate.

SUPER-CARBONATIS POTASSAE, AQUA: Solution of LIXIVA supersaturated with FIXED AIR. Lithontriptic. [23]

SUPER-CARBONATIS SODAE: Sodium bicarbonate.

SUPER-CARBONATIS SODAE, AQUA: Solution of BARILLA supersaturated with FIXED AIR. Lithontriptic. [23]

SUPER-SULPHAS ALUMINAE ET POTASSAE [EXSICCATUS]: Same as ALUM.

SUPER-TARTRIS POTASSAE: Same as CREAM OF TARTAR.

Supplantiva, Elixir: An unguent applied to the soles of the feet, to draw noxious materials down and out of the body.

Suppository: A remedy designed for insertion into the rectum; often made with salt and honey. Prescribed when the patient "cannot be put into a suitable posture of body, to receive a glyster, or when a glyster is not likely to be retained long enough to be of any service." [12]

SUPPURATIVUM, UNGUENTUM: 1) Same as BASILICON OINTMENT. 2) A sparadrapum.

SUS ADEPS: Same as AXUNGUENTUM PORCINUM.

SWAIM'S PANACEA: Invented about 1820 by William Swaim of Philadelphia, it was made with SARSAPARILLA, GAULTHERIA, and HYDRARGYRUS MURIATUS CORROSIVUS, and promoted as a blood purifier for the cure of scrofula, syphilis, mercury toxicity, and rheumatism. By 1830, SENNA, SASSAFRAS, flowers of BORAGO, leaves of ROSAE, and marsh grass had been added to the original formula.

SWALLOW WORT: See VINCETOXICUM.

SWALLOWS, OIL OF: See HIRUNDINUM.

SWEET FLAG: See CALAMUS AROMATICUS.

SWIETENIA: See SOYMIDA.

SYDENHAM'S LAUDANUM: see LAUDANUM, SYDENHAM'S.

SYDENHAM'S PLASTER: A poultice made of MICA PANIO, CROCUS, and OL ROSARUM. Attributed to 17th-century English physician Thomas Sydenham of London.

SYLVIUS, [CARMINATIVE] SPIRIT OF: A preparation of SPIRITUS AMMONIAE invented about 1650 by Dr. Franz de la Boë of Leyden, also called Franciscus Sylvius.

SYLVIUS, FEVER (or DIGESTIVE) SALT OF: Same as SPIRIT OF SYLVIUS.

SYMPATHETIC OINTMENT OF PARACELSUS: Made, in the autumn, of powdered burnt worms, dried boar's brain, red sandalwood, powdered mummy, bloodstone, moss from the skull of a man who had died a violent death (preferably by hanging, and if he had not been buried; it should be collected at moonrise, preferably under Venus), and a mixture of boar's and bear's fat. This "sympathetic" medicine for treating wound victims is to be applied to the instrument that had inflicted the wound, not to the patient, although his wound was to be cleaned and dressed daily. [13; also see any edition of Oliver Wendell Holmes' essay on "Homeopathy and its Kindred Delusions"]

SYMPATHETIC POWDER: 1) A powder that effected a cure if anything soaked with blood of the injured person were immersed in a solution of the powder. [See Lester S. King, *The Road to Medical Enlightenment* (London: Macdonald, 1970), pp. 140-145, and any edition of Oliver Wendell Holmes' essay on "Homeopathy and Its Kindred Delusions"] 2) Powdered ZINCUM VITRIOLATUM that has been exposed to the sun under the sign of Leo in July; perhaps same material as in def. no. 1.

SYMPHYTUM: Same as CONSOLIDA.

SYMPLOCARPUS: See ARUM AMERICANUM.

Synanchica: Sore throat remedies.

Syncoptica: Remedies for fainting.

Syncritica: Remedies that relax the body.

Synulotica: Remedies for cicatrizing wounds.

Syringe: An animal bladder, or a metal tube with a piston, used for injecting fluids into the rectum (i.e., enemas), vagina, or urethra.

Syrup: A drug preparation made by mixing the raw ingredients in simple syrup or honey.

SYRUPUS EMPYREUMATICUS: "Foul-tasting syrup," blackstrap molasses, which has a high sulfur content.

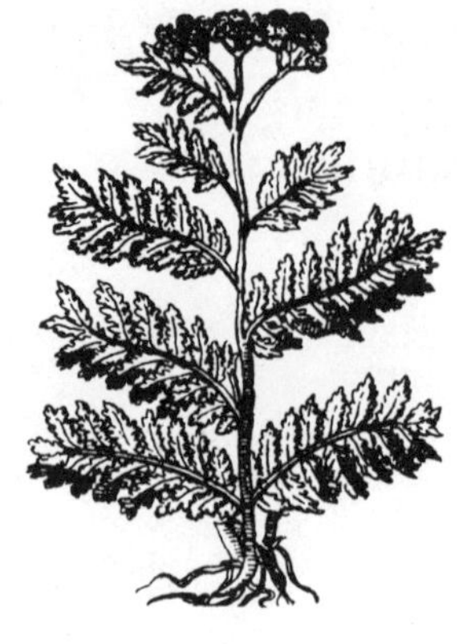

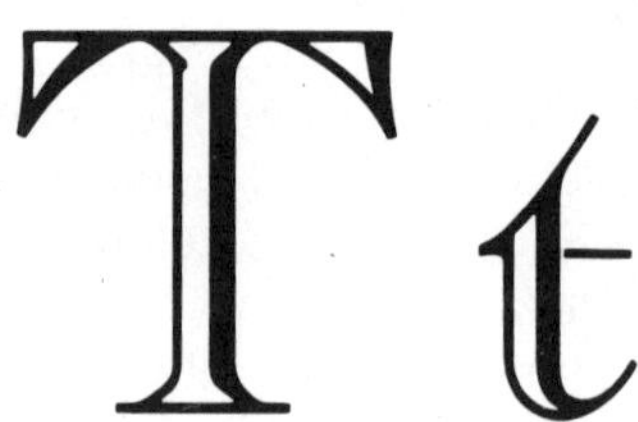

Tanacetum

TABACUM: Same as NICOTIANA.

Tabellae: Tablets or lozenges.

TACAMAHACA: Resin of tacamahaca, or Carolina poplar, *Populus balsamifera* (but sometimes South American species such as *Fagara octandra* were used). Said to be used by American Indians for softening superficial tumors and for limb pains; also, diuretic and antiscorbutic. [15]

TAGETES: See CALENDULA.

TAMARINDORUM CUM SENNA, INFUSUM: "Infusion of tamarinds with senna," a water extract of TAMARINDUS, SENNA, CREAM OF TARTAR, CORIANDRUM, and SACCHARUM NON PURIFICATUM, and mixed in a non-leaden vessel to avoid lead poisoning. Mild cooling cathartic. [1,15]

TAMARINDUS [INDICA]: Fruits of tamarind, *Tamarindus indica*. Acid cathartic with refrigerant and thirst-quenching properties. [15,23,29,30]

TAME POISON: See VINCETOXICUM.

TANACETUM [VULGARE]: Flowers, leaves, or seeds of tansy, *Tanacetum vulgare*. Antihysteric, deobstruent, tonic, emmenagogue, anthelminthic, and gout preventive.

[15,23,2930] Contains thujone, for which see ABSINTHUM.

TANSY: See TANACETUM.

TAR: Same as PIX LIQUIDA.

TARAXACUM: Root and leaves of dandelion, *Taraxacum officinale*. Tonic, aperient, and diuretic (hence its French name, *pisse-en-lit*), especially in dropsy. [15,23,29]

TARTAR: See CREAM OF TARTAR.

TARTAR EMETIC: Same as ANTIMONIUM TARTARISATUM.

TARTARI, CRYSTALLI: Crystalline form of CREAM OF TARTAR.

TARTARICUM, ACIDUM: Tartaric acid. Used as a cheap substitute for ACIDUM CITRICUM, and in making soda powders, e.g., SEIDLITZ POWDERS.

TARTARIFIED SODA: Same as CREAM OF TARTAR.

TARTARI, SAL: "Salt of tartar," potassium tartrate. Used as a diuretic, as a mild cooling cathartic especially suitable for mental patients, and as a strong cathartic, depending on dose. [1,15,23]

TARTARIS ANTIMONIAE: Same as ANTIMONIUM TARTARISATUM.

TARTARUM REGENERATUM: Same as LIXIVA ACETATA.

TARTARUS EMETICUS: Same as ANTIMONIUM TARTARISATUM.

TARTARUS STIBIATUS: Same as ANTIMONIUM TARTARISATUM.

TARTARUS VITRIOLATUS: Same as KALI SULPHURATUM.

TARTRIS POTASSAE: Same as SAL TARTARI.

TARTRIS POTASSAE ET SODAE: Same as CREAM OF TARTAR.

TAR WATER: See BERKELEY'S TAR WATER.

TASTELESS AGUE DROPS: Nearly same as SOLUTIO ARSENICI MINERALIS.

TEA: See THEA.

TELA GUALTERI: "Gaultier's web," a sparadrapum.

Tentipellium: A remedy for smoothing skin wrinkles.

TEREBINTHA ARGENTORATENSIS: "Strasbourg turpentine," made from an unidentified botanical source. Properties like those of TEREBINTHA VENETA. [15]

TEREBINTHA [VENETA], OL: Turpentine, the volatile oil(s)

extracted and distilled chiefly from *Pinus sylvestris* (Scotch pine) in Europe, *Larix caricina* or *L. decidua* in the northern American states, *P. palustris* and *P. taeda* in the southern American states, and *Abies balsamea* in Canada. Given internally, but seldom, as a stimulating diuretic, diaphoretic, and, because of its detergent activity, as a gentle cathartic (and anthelminthic); most often applied externally in unguents and liniments, and as a styptic for nose bleeds. Makes urine smell like violets. [1,2,15,23,29,30; also see John S. Haller, Jr., "Sampson of the Terebinthates: Medical History of Turpentine," *Southern Medical Journal* 77 (1984): 750-754] Turpentine and one of its extracts, terpin hydrate, are still used as expectorants.

TEREBINTHA VULGARIS: Common turpentine, distilled from resins from *Pinus* or *Abies* spp. Although this preparation has medical properties like those of OL TEREBINTHA, it is so crude that it is used chiefly only in plasters and ointments. [15]

TERRA DAMNATA: "Condemned earth." Same as CAPUT MORTUUM.

TERRA DULCIS VITRIOLI: Thoroughly washed FERRUM VITRIOLATUM. Astringent.

TERRA FOLIATA TARTARI: Same as LIXIVA ACETATA.

TERRA JAPONICA: Same as CATECHU.

TERRA LEMNIA: See LEMNIAN EARTH.

TERRA SIGILLATA: A generic term for many different earth tablets, e.g., SILESIAN EARTH, each bearing a distinctive seal attesting to its place of origin.

TERRA SILESIANA: Same as SILESIAN EARTH.

TESTACEOUS CERATA, PULVIS: A mixture of CERATE and OSTREA EDULIS.

Testaceous Powder: One made with OSTREA EDULIS.

TEUCRIUM: See CHAMAEDRYS, MARUM SYRIACUM, and SCORDIUM.

THAPSIA: Deadly carrot, *Thapsia garganica*. Emetic and cathartic. Also see SILPHIUM.

THAPSUS BARBATUS: Same as VERBASCUM.

THEA: Leaf of tea, *Thea sinensis*. First brought to Europe in 1610, it slowly gained popularity as a tonic beverage over the next 40 years. Diluent, diuretic, and diaphoretic; causes weakness and tremors in high doses; however, most of its effects are attributable simply to the warm water in which it is taken. [15] Theophylline, now a mainstay of treatment for asthma, was discovered in tea by A. Kossel in 1888, but caffeine (see COFFEA) is far more abundant in tea leaves.

THEBAIC [OPIUM]: 1) The best quality OPIUM, which came from Thebes (modern Luxor), Egypt. 2) Synonym for any OPIUM preparation.

THEBAICA, TINCTURA: Made by letting 2 oz. OPIUM stand in two pints PROOF SPIRIT for four days and then straining and evaporating until one drachm of tincture contained 3½ grains of pure opium; aromatic spices were sometimes added. [1,2,3,23]

THEBAIC ELECTUARY: Same as ELECTUARIUM OPIATUM.

THEBAIC PILL: 1) A mixture of OPIUM, GLYCERRHIZA, and soap; sometimes PIMENTO was added to "correct" the opium by preventing its "bad effects." A ten-grain pill should contain one grain of opium. Another stronger formulation included OPIUM, CAMPHOR, and soap. [1,3,15,23] 2) Any OPIUM pill.

THEBAICUM, ELECTUARIUM: Same as ELECTUARIUM OPIATUM.

THEBAICUM, INFUSUM: A water solution of OPIUM, often with added CATECHU. Probably because the active principles of opium are less soluble in water than in alcohol, this preparation was prescribed less often than TINCTURA THEBAICA, which was more potent and more predictable. [1,3]

THEBAICUM, UNGUENTUM: Same as LINIMENTUM OPIATUM.

THEBAICUS, PULVIS: Powder of OPIUM and NITER, the latter to ameliorate the warming properties of the opium. [15]

THEOBROMA: See CACOA.

THERIAC: An OPIUM preparation (said to have been devised as a modification of MITHRIDATE by Andromachus, physician to the emperor Nero) that contained over 50 ingredients. It included 2.5-15.2 mg. morphine per recommended dose, depending on body weight. Narcotic. A formula published in Edinburgh in 1794 included: Troches of squills, long pepper, strained opium, dried vipers, cinnamon, opobalsam (or oil of nutmeg), agaric, Florence orris root, scordium, red roses, navew seeds, liquorice, Indian nard, saffron, amomum, myrrh, costus (or zedoary), camel's hay, cinquefoil root, rhubarb, ginger, Indian leaf (or mace), dittany of Crete, horehound leaves, calamint, stechas, black pepper, Macedonian parsley seed, olibanum, Chio turpentine, valerian, gentian, Celtic nard, spignel, poley mountain, St. John's wort, groundpine, germander tops with seed, carpobalsam (or cubebs), anise seed, sweet fennel seed, lesser cardamon seeds, bishop's weed, hartwort, treacle mustard, hypocistis, acacia (or Japan earth), gum arabic, storax, sagapenum, terra lemnia (or bole armenic or French bole), green vitriol, small (or long) birthwort root, lesser centaury tops, candy carrot seed, opopanax, galbanum, castor, Jews pitch (or white amber), calamus aromaticus, and clarified honey. [2,3,15] These 61 ingredients include many of the 45 used to make MITHRIDATE. The Rev. Thomas Harward of Boston proposed a simplified method for preparing this exemplar of polypharmacy in the first book on any drug to be published in America (1732). [See Glenn Sonnedecker, "Harward's *Electuarium* . . . Earliest Drug Treatise Published by an American Colonist?," *Pharmacy in History 19* (1977), 24-38; also see Gilbert Watson, *Theriac and Mithradatium* (London: Wellcome Historical Medical Library, 1966)]

THERIACA ANDROMACHI: Essentially, same as THERIAC or VENICE TREACLE.

THERIACA EDINENSIS: An abbreviated formula of THERIAC introduced in the 1722 Edinburgh *Pharmacopoeia*, it was made of ANGELICA, CAMPHOR, CONTRAYERVA, COSTUS, CROCUS, GUIAC, LAURUS, MYRRH, OPIUM, RUTA, SCORDIUM, SERPENTINA, VALERIANA, an aromatic powder (probably PULVIS AROMATICUS), honey, and enough wine to dissolve the opium. CASTOREUM was added in 1744, but in 1774 this formula was replaced by that for ELECTUARIUM OPIATUM.

THERIACA LONDINENSIS: Nearly same as THERIACA EDINENSIS.

Thermantica: Warming remedies.

THISTLE, BASTARD SAFFRON: See CARTHAMUS.

THISTLE, YELLOW: See ARGEMONE MEXICANA.

THOMPSON'S PANACEA: A 1705 proprietary formula that contained HYDRARGYRUS PURIFICATUS, SULPHUR, and a salt of ANTIMONIUM. Antivenereal.

THORN APPLE: See STRAMONIUM.

THOROUGH WORT: See EUPATORIUM entries.

THRIDAX: Juice of LACTUCA, used as a sedative; probably same as LACTUCARIUM.

THURIS COMPOSITUM, EMPLASTRUM: "Compound plaster of frankincense," a tonic and astringent plaster made with THUS, SANGUIS DRACONIS, and WHITE LEAD; especially suitable for children. [15]

THUS: Common "frankincense," a brittle resin from pine species that also produce TEREBINTHA VULGARIS. Used chiefly in plasters. [15] For true frankincense, see OLIBANUM.

THUS MASCULUM, FAEMININUM, or CORTICOSUM: Forms of OLIBANUM.

THYMUS: Common thyme, *Thymus vulgaris*. Aromatic; analgesic for toothache. [15] Thymol, or camphor of thyme, was isolated in 1719 by Kaspar Neumann, court apothecary at Berlin; thymol was used until recently as an antimicrobial agent and in a test for assessing liver function.

TIGLII, OLEUM: Croton oil, from seeds of *Croton tiglium*; introduced from India to England about 1812. A rapidly acting potent hydragogue cathartic. Side effects include vomiting, severe abdominal pain, and death. [29,30]

TILIA: Flowers of linden (sometimes also called lime in the 18th century) tree, *Tilia europea* or other spp. Antiepileptic, antispasmodic. [15]

TILLY DROPS: Same as DUTCH DROPS.

TINCAL: Same as BORAX.

Tincture: An alcohol solution of a non-volatile drug ingredient.

TINKER'S-WEED: See TRIOSTEUM.

Tisane: Same as Ptisan.

TOAD-FLAX: See LINARIA.

TOBACCO: See NICOTIANA.

TOLUIFERA BALSAMUM: Same as BALSAM OF PERU.

TOLU, BALSAM or SYRUP OF: Resin of *Myroxylon balsamum*, a South American drug first described by Dr. Nicolas Monardes of Seville in 1574. Tonic and weak expectorant. [15,23,29,30]

TOLUTANUM: Same as SYRUP OF TOLU.

Tonic: A drug that strengthens the body, via the stomach, by increasing the force of the circulation, animal heat, secretions, digestion, or muscular action. Vegetable tonics are more potent than mineral products. Used to treat debilitating conditions. By the mid-19th century, tonics were thought to increase the body's energy generally, rather than to be selective for some one function, such as urine output or sweating, more than others.

TOOTHACHE TREE: See ARALIA SPINOSA.

TORCULARIA: Literally, "wine presses." Tourniquets, sometimes applied in rotation from limb to limb, to facilitate redistribution of edema fluid. [1]

TORMENTILLA [ERECTA]: Root of tormentil, or septfoil, *Potentilla erecta* (or *P. tormentilla*). Astringent. [2,23,29]

TORMENTORIUS, PULVIS: "Artillery powder," i.e., gunpowder, made with NITER, CHARCOAL, and SULPHUR. Also see PULVIS FULMINANS.

Toxica: Poisons.

TOXICODENDRON: See RHUS entries.

Trachea: Sharp, irritating, and ulcerating remedies.

TRAGACANTH, GUM: Extract of *Astragalus gummifer*. Used to increase the viscosity of liquid drugs, and as a demulcent. [2,23,29,30] Still used for similar purposes.

TRAGEA GRANORUM ACTES: "Elder seed troches," made with EBULUS and RYE flour. Antidysenteric.

TRAGEA MERCURIALIS: "Mercury troches," a panacea made with HYDRARGYRUS and GUM TRAGACANTH.

TRANQUILLE, BAUME: A panacea invented by a Capuchin monk, Father Tranquille, in the 17th century. It contained 20 ingredients, including OPIUM, NICOTIANA, STRAMONIUM, ABSINTHUM, LAVANDULA, and RUTA. [13]

TRANQUILLE, SEL: "Tranquillizing salt," SAL SEDATUM.

TRAUMATICUM, BALSAMUM: "Wound balsam." Same as TURLINGTON'S BALSAM, q.v.

TREACLE: See VENICE TREACLE.

TRIBUS, MIXTURA DE: "Three-part mixture," made with THERIAC (with added CAMPHOR), VITRIOL, and SAL TARTARI.

TRICHOMANES: Common, or English, maidenhair fern, *Asplenium trichomanes*. Expectorant and deobstruent. [15]

TRIFOLIUM PALUDOSUM: Leaves of buck-bean, or marsh trefoil, *Menyanthes trifoliata*. Aperient, deobstruent, stomachic, diuretic, and diaphoretic; emetic in large doses. [15,29,30]

Trigona: Narcotic remedies.

TRIGONELLA: See FENUGREEK.

TRIOSTEUM: Root of fever-root, feverwort, or tinker's weed, *Triosteum perfoliatum*. Cathartic and diuretic; emetic in large doses. [29,30]

TRITICUM [AESTIVUM or HYBERNUM]: Flour and starch from wheat, *Triticum aestivum*. Used to thicken compound medicines, as a nutriment, and as a visceral tonic. [15] Also see GRAMEN.

Troche: A powder made up with glutinous materials (e.g., GUM ARABIC and GUM TRAGACANTH) into little cakes and then dried. Used chiefly to permit slow release of the active materials into the stomach.

Troschici: Troches.

TROSCHICI BECHICI: See BECHICI TROSCHICI.

TROUT-LILY: See ERYTHRONIUM.

Troy Weights: See Measurement.

TULIP TREE: See LIRIODENDRON TULIPIFERA.

TURBITH: See TURPETHUM.

TURKS, WINE OF THE: Same as LAUDANUM; its OPIUM content was imported from Ottoman-ruled Egypt (see THEBAIC).

TURLINGTON'S BALSAM OF LIFE: Patented by Robert Turlington in 1744, it was made of 27 ingredients and said to cure urinary tract stones, colic, and "inward weakness;" later advertisements promoted it simply as a panacea. A 20th-century formula included BENZOIN, STYRAX CALAMITA, BALSAM OF TOLU, BALSAM OF PERU, ALOES, MYRRH, and ANGELICA. Became official as BALSAMUM TRAUMATICUM in 1746, and later as TINCTURA BENZOINI COMPOSITA. [14]

TURMERIC: 1) Usually, same as CURCUMA. 2) Sometimes, in U.S., same as SANGUINARIA CANADENSIS.

TURNER'S CERATE: An unguent made with CALAMINE, CERA FLAVA, OL OLIVA, and unsalted butter; devised by "Dr." Daniel Turner of London in the early 18th century.

TURPENTINE: See TEREBINTHA entries.

TURPETH (or TURBITH) MINERALIS: Same as HYDRARGYRUS VITRIOLATUS; Dr. Oswald Croll of Anhalt, a Paracelsian chemist, coined this term in the 16th century to indicate the salt's physical resemblance to TURPETHUM. (Actually, it was mercuric subsulfate, $HgSO_4 \cdot 2H_2O$.)

TURPETHUM: Bark of root of turbith, *Ipomoea turpethum*, a

vine related to JALAP. Undependable and unsafe cathartic. [15]

TUSSILAGO [FARFARI]: Leaves and flowers of colt's foot, *Tussilago farfara*. Demulcent expectorant. [15,23,29]

TUSSIVUM, UNGUENTUM: "Cough ointment." Same as LINIMENTUM AMMONIAE.

TUTIAE, UNGUENT: Impure ZINCUM USTUM mixed with lead or copper oxides, in an appropriate base (the original formula called for viper fat). "Tutiae" is a Latinization of an unknown word perhaps of Sanskrit origin. Emollient used in unguents and collyria. [2,15]

TUTTY: Probably the original form of TUTIAE.

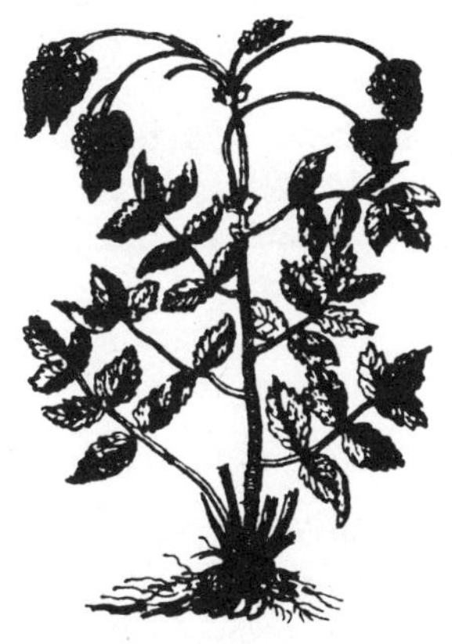

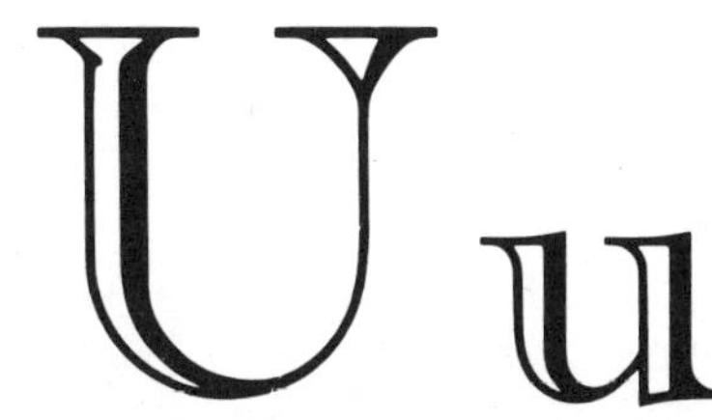

Ulmaria

ULMARIA: Root of European meadowsweet, *Spiraea ulmaria* or, in U.S., *S. latifolia* (neither should be confused with English meadowsweet, *Filipendula ulmaria*). Used in some plasters, but with no specific medicinal effect of its own. [15] However, also see SALIX.

ULMUS: Fresh inner bark of elm tree, *Ulmus campestris*. Demulcent, diuretic, and an astringent for chronic skin conditions. [15,29]

ULMUS RUBRA: Red, or slippery, elm, *Ulmus rubra*. Emollient, diet drink, expectorant, antidiarrheal, and a demulcent wound dressing. [23,29,30]

Umbel plaster: One that surrounds a limb.

UNCARIA: See CATECHU.

Uncia: Ounce; see Measurement.

Unguent: A plaster that has been diluted with oil to the consistency of stiff honey.

UNGUENTUM SIMPLEX: Simple ointment; made of five parts OL OLIVA and two parts CERA ALBA. Used for dressing wounds and skin sores. [1,2]

UNIVERSALIS, CONFECTIO: A panacea electuary of unknown composition.

URGINEA: See SCILLA.

URINALIS, HERBA: Same as LINARIA.

URTICA [DIOICA]: Leaves of common nettle, *Urtica dioica*. Powerful rubefacient, stimulant, febrifuge, and lithontriptic. [15,23]

UTERINUM, ELIXIR: "Uterine elixir." Same as TINCTURA SABINAE COMPOSITA.

UTERINUM, TINCTURA: "Uterine tincture." Made with MYRRH, CROCUS, CASTOR, CAMPHOR, HARTSHORN, and VINUM. Antihysteric and emmenagogue.

UVA[E] PASSA[E]: 1) Currants, dried grapes of *Vitis corinthiaca*. For flavoring. [15] 2) Raisins, sun-dried grapes of *Vitis damascena*. Used in several drug mixtures, but for no specific medicinal effect, [15] although raisins were often said to produce catharsis. [2,29]

UVA URSI: Leaves of bearberry, wild cranberry, or whortleberry, *Arctostaphylos uva-ursi*. Introduced to medical practice in 1763 in Berlin by Dr. Karl Abraham Gerhard. Astringent, nephritic, and a visceral tonic. [2,15,29,30]

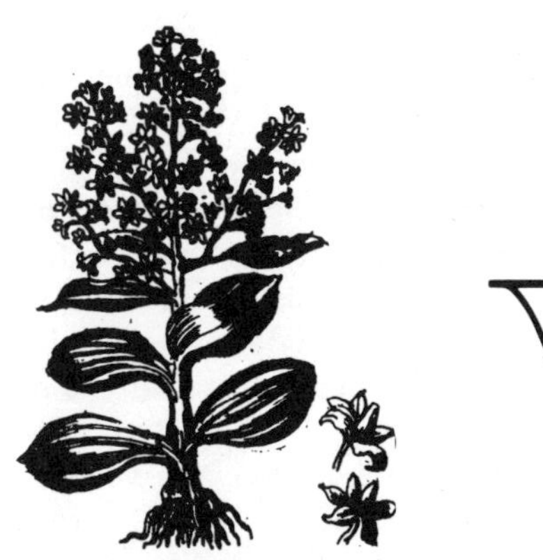

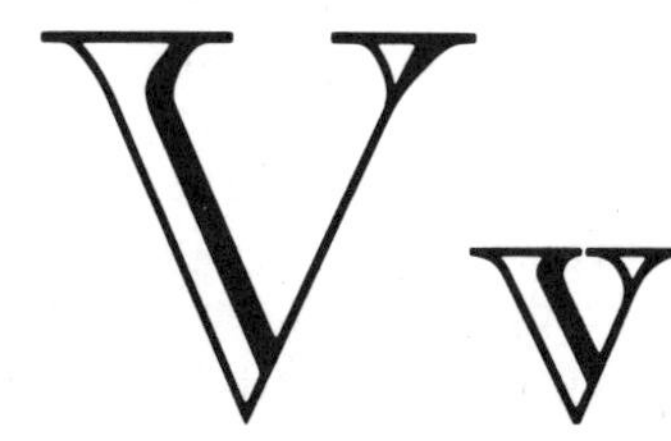

Veratrum album

VALERIANA SYLVESTRIS (or OFFICINALIS): Root of valerian, or garden-heliotrope, *Valeriana officinalis*. Tonic, antiepileptic, antispasmodic, antihysteric, anodyne, and soporific. [1,2,15,23,29,30] A weak sedative.

VAN SWIETEN, BARK: A preparation of CINCHONA introduced by Dr. Gerhard van Swieten of Vienna about 1750. [1]

VAN SWIETEN'S ANTIVENEREAL: Same as HYDRARGYRUS MURIATUS CORROSIVUS. Promoted by Dr. Gerhard van Swieten of Vienna about 1750. [2]

Vectiaria: Violent cathartics.

VEGETABLE ACID, POTUS: Most often, an infusion of LIXIVA. However, sometimes it was prepared as CREAM OF TARTAR dissolved in flour and water. Relieves thirst, and stimulates weak stomachs. [1]

VEGETABLE ALKALI, FIXED: Same as LIXIVA.

VEGETO-MINERAL WATER: Same as GOULARD'S EXTRACT OF SATURN.

VENICE TREACLE: A preparation much like THERIAC, containing 1.3% OPIUM, which provided 2.5-15.2 mg. morphine per recommended dose, depending on body weight, as well as SCILLA and about 57 other ingredients. [3,13]

VERATRUM ALBUM: Root of white hellebore, *Veratrum album*. Violent emetic; strong, perhaps unsafe, errhine; convulsant; also applied topically to skin eruptions. [15,23,29] In 1819, French chemists Pierre-Joseph Pelletier and Joseph-Bienaimée Caventou isolated its active principle, veratrine (actually several "veratrine alkaloids").

VERATRUM VIRIDE: Rhizome of American or false hellebore, Indian poke, poke root, or swamp hellebore, *Veratrum viride*. In 1673 the English Traveller John Josselyn reported that New England Indians used it in ordeals by emesis. Resembles HELLEBORUS ALBUS in its effects, especially vomiting, but less potent as a cathartic; diuretic and diaphoretic, and sometimes used to treat gout. Side effects include bradycardia, faintness, mydriasis, dim vision, vertigo, and headache. [29,30] The active principle, veratrine (actually several "veratrine alkaloids"), was isolated from it by K. F. W. Meissner of Halle in 1818. Although veratrine can reduce blood pressure, its toxicity precludes its clinical use as an antihypertensive agent.

VERBASCUM: Leaf of mullein, *Verbascum thapsis*. Antitussive and diaphoretic; an emollient for lung or intestinal disorders; perhaps anodyne; also applied topically to skin ulcers. [15,29]

VERDEGRIS or VERDIGRIS: Literally, "Green [substance] from Greece." Copper acetate. Escharotic, for surgical dressings; sometimes used as a potent emetic. [2,8,15,23,29,30]

VERONICA: See BECCABUNGA.

Vesicatorium: A blister.

VESSICATIVUM, TINCTURA: "Blistering tincture," usually TINCTURA CANTHARIDIS.

VICIA FABA: See FABA.

VIE, BAUME DE: "Balm of life," invented in the 18th century by a French apothecary named Le Lievre. Made with Socotrine ALOES, GENTIANA, RHEI, VENICE TREACLE, CROCUS, AGARICUS, ZEDOARIA, MYRRH, PROOF SPIRIT, and sugar. Recommended as a tonic that does not increase body heat. [13] However, many other identically-named formulas were widely available.

VIGANI'S VOLATILE ELIXIR OF VITRIOL: A proprietary formulation of VITRIOLICI AROMATICUS, SPIRITUS AETHERIS.

VIGO[NIUM], EMPLASTRUM: A complex mercurial plaster devised about 1500 by Dr. Giovanni di Vigo of Rome, it was made with earthworms, frogs, viper's flesh (or human fat), wine, CAMEL'S HAY, LAVENDULA, CHAMAEMELUM, WHITE LEAD, and HYDRARGYRUS PURIFICATUS, and several aromatic ingredients. Antisyphilitic. [13]

VINAIGRE DES QUATRE VOLEURS: "Vinegar of the Four Thieves." During a plague at Toulouse in 1628, four men are said to have used this medicine successfully to protect themselves while robbing the sick and dead under the pretence of treating them. One of the thieves was caught, but saved himself from the gallows by revealing the ingredients of the prophylactic vinegar, hence this name for it. The original formula was made with RUTA, ROSMARINUS, MENTHA PIPERITA, and ABSINTHUM. It became more complex over the next century, especially as the formula prepared at Marseilles, but by the late 18th century it was the same as ACETUM AROMATICUM (q.v.). [15, p. 466]

VINCETOXICUM: Root of swallow wort, or tame poison (literally, "antipoison"), *Vincetoxicum officinal* or *V. asclepiadea*. Diaphoretic, diuretic, emmenagogue, and alexipharmic; similar to VALERIANA. [15]

VINEGAR: See ACETUM.

VINI GALLICI, SPIRITUS: "Spirit of French wine." Brandy.

VINI, OLEUM: "Oil of wine," nearly same as AETHER VITRIOLICUS, but made by distilling the ALCOHOL and VITRIOL over potassium.

VINOSUS RECTIFICATUS [sive PURISSIMUS], SPIRITUS: "Rectified spirit of wine," containing 95% alcohol, with a specific gravity of 0.8333 or 0.835. A common menstruum. Because it coagulates all animal fluids except urine, and hardens solid tissues, it can be applied externally to strengthen blood vessels and prevent hemorrhage. Because it inhibits sensory and motor activity when applied topically to nerves in small doses, it can raise the spirits and promote agility, and in large doses destroys voluntary motion and produces intoxication. In even larger doses, it destroys the lining of the stomach, and causes death in palsy or apoplexy. [15] Also see ALCOHOL and VINUM.

Vinum: A strained solution of active drug material(s) in wine.

VINUM: Fermented juice of grapes. In late 18th-century Britain, four varieties were used as menstrua for extracting drugs: *Vinum album Hispanicum*, mountain wine; *Vinum Canarium*, Canary wine or sack; *Vinum Rhenanum*, Rhine wine; and *Vinum rubrum*, red port. They differed chiefly in the amounts of water, tartar, gummy resinous astringent matter (including the coloring), and, especially, alcohol, contained in each. (For the alcohol content of different wines, see ref. 29, pp. 739-740, and ref. 30, pp. 392-393). The therapeutic goals of wine are: "to stimulate the stomach, cheer the spirits, warm the habit, promote perspiration, render the vessels full and turgid, raise the pulse, and quicken the circulation." Digestive; stimulates the heart and arteries; raises body heat. In short, the major effect of wine is tonic, largely because it is astringent. [15,29,30] Also see ALCOHOL and SPIRITUS VINOSUS RECTIFICATUS.

VIOLA [ODORATA]: Fresh flowers of violets, *Viola odorata*. A gentle cathartic especially suitable for children; also, an emollient expectorant and nephritic. [15,29]

VIOLARUM, TABELLAE DE SUCCO: "Violet juice tablets." A cathartic electuary based on VIOLA juice.

VIPERA: Flesh of Britain's only venomous snake, *Pelias berus*. A nutritious restorative; heats and dries by increasing thirst; also applied to chronic skin conditions. [15; 39, pp. 316-318]

VIRGA AUREA: In Europe, leaves of goldenrod, *Solidago virgaurea*. Astringent tonic, carminative, and diaphoretic. [15,29,30] Also see SOLIDAGO.

VIRGINIA SNAKEROOT: See SERPENTARIA.

VIRGIN'S-BOWER: See FLAMULA JOVIS.

VIRIDEM, BALSAM: "Green balsam," made with VERDEGRIS.

VISCUS: Wood of mistletoe, *Loranthus europaeus* (but possibly *Viscus albus*) in Europe, and *Phoradendron flavescens* in North America. Once worn around the neck to prevent witchcraft and taken internally to expel poisons. Antispasmodic. [15]

VITIS: Leaves and stems of the grape, *Vitis vinifera*. Astringent, anti-inflammatory, and diuretic. [15]

VITIS VINIFERA: 1) VINUM. 2) Raisins; see UVA PASSA.

VITRIFIED ANTIMONY: Same as ANTIMONIUM VITRIFICATUM.

VITRIOL [OL]: Sulfuric acid. Used topically, after dilution

with seven or eight parts of water, as a caustic and rubefacient, and internally as an astringent antiseptic, refrigerant, stomachic, or tonic. [15,23,29] Also see entries beginning with SULPHUR.

VITRIOL ANTIMONIUM: Sulfurated antimony. Emetic and cathartic. [2] Also see KERMES MINERALE.

VITRIOLATED SODA: Sodium sulfate. Cathartic and diuretic. [23,29,30]

VITRIOLATED TARTAR: Same as KALI SULPHURATUM.

VITRIOLATUM CALCINATUM: Same as FERRUM VITRIOLATUM EXSICCATUM.

VITRIOLATUM SULPHURATUM LIXIVA: Same as KALI SULPHURATUM.

VITRIOL, BLUE: Copper sulfate. Astringent and tonic when taken by mouth (but vomiting is a frequent side effect); escharotic when applied topically. [23,29]

VITRIOL, ELIXIR [OF]: Same as ACIDUM VITRIOLI AROMATICUM.

VITRIOLI ACIDUM, ELIXIR: Same as VITRIOLI AROMATICUM, ACIDUM.

VITRIOLI AROMATICUM, ACIDUM: "Aromatic acid of vitriol," made of VITRIOL in wine, CINNAMOMUM, and ZINGIBER. Tonic, astringent, and stomachic, especially when the body has been weakened by fever. [2,15,29]

VITRIOLIC ETHER: Same as AETHER VITRIOLICUS.

VITRIOLICI AROMATICUS, SPIRITUS AETHERIS: "Aromatic spirit of vitriolic ether," made with CINNAMOMUM, CARDAMOMUM MINUS, PIPER LONGUM, and ANGELICA, as in TINCTURA AROMATICA, but in AETHER VITRIOLICUS instead of alcohol. Mild tonic. [15]

VITRIOLICUM DILUTUM, ACIDUM: "Dilute vitriolic acid;" made of one part VITRIOL, at specific gravity 1.85, and seven parts of water, at Edinburgh (one and nine parts, respectively, at London). Its effects are those of VITRIOL.

VITRIOLICUM, LINIMENTUM, or UNGUENTUM: Made with one part of ACIDUM VITRIOLICUM DILUTUM and eight parts of OL OLIVA. Used as a rubefacient, and to counteract the effect of HYDRARGYRUS on the gums. [1,15]

VITRIOLICUS, AETHER: "Sulphuric ether" (now called

ethyl ether or diethyl ether), prepared by distilling equal parts of VITRIOL and VINUM together. Introduced by Valerius Cordus in 1540 (although Paracelsus may have described its preparation and effects 15 years earlier). Taken internally as a diaphoretic, diuretic, antispasmodic, tonic, analgesic, and narcotic; applied externally as a stimulating rubefacient that, paradoxically, produces a sensation of cold. Also used to dissolve elastic gums for making adhesive plasters. The vitriolic component is more important therapeutically than the etheric component (although no sulfur atoms are present in ether). [1,13,23,29,30] The true chemical formula of ether was established by Charles Gerhardt in 1842. Dr. Crawford W. Long of Jefferson, Georgia, operated on patients under ether anesthesia in 1842-1845, but did not publish until 1849, three years after dentist William T. G. Morton and surgeon John C. Warren had given the first public demonstration of ether's efficacy in producing surgical anesthesia at Boston's Massachusetts General Hospital.

VITRIOLI DULCIS, SPIRITUS: Same as AETHER VITRIOLICUS.

VITRIOL OF HEAVY EARTH: Barium sulfate.

VITRIOL, OL: Same as VITRIOL.

VITRIOL ROMANUM: Same as VITRIOL, BLUE.

VITRIOLUM ALBUM: Same as ZINCUM VITRIOLATUM.

VITRIOLUM CAERULEUM: Same as VITRIOL, BLUE.

VITRIOLUM VIRIDE: Same as FERRUM VITRIOLATUM.

VITRIOL, WHITE: Same as ZINCUM VITRIOLATUM.

VIVIFICANTES IMPERIALES, TABELLAE: "Royal tablets of longevity," a heart stimulant made with CONFECTIO KERMES.

VOLATILE ALKALI: Same as SPIRITUS AMMONIAE.

VOLATILE DROPS (or SALTS): 1) SPIRITUS AMMONIAE AROMATICUS or AQUA AMMONIAE. 2) AMMONIA PRAEPARATA. Antispasmodic and tonic; often used as smelling salts. 3) Other "volatile" medicines included CAJEPUT, CAMPHOR, SAL AMMONIAC, SAL TARTARI (or ACIDUM TARTARICUM), and VOLATILE ALKALI. [2]

VOLATILE, LINIMENT: Same as LINIMENTUM AMMONIAE.

VOLATILE OLEOSUM, SAL: Same as SPIRITUS AMMONIAE AROMATICUS.
V.S.: Abbreviation for venesection; see BLEEDING.
Vulnerary: A medicine that promotes wound healing.

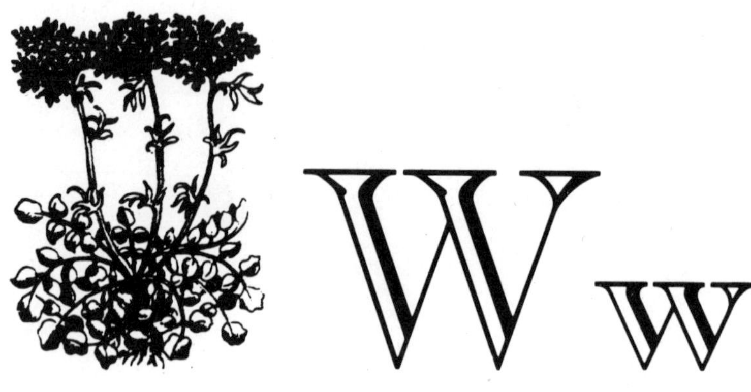

Watercress

WADE'S BALSAM: A proprietary liniment much like TINCTURA BENZOINI COMPOSITA.

WAKE ROBIN: See ARUM MACULATUM.

WALLWORT: Same as URTICA.

WALNUT: See JUGLANS CINEREA.

WARD'S DROPS: Devised by Joshua ("Spot") Ward, a famous London "quack," in the early 18th century, it was ANTIMONIUM VITRIFICATUM dissolved in Malaga wine. [13]

WARD'S DROPSY PURGING POWDER: Devised by Joshua Ward, it was made of JALAP, CREAM OF TARTAR, and IRIS FLORENTINA (later replaced by BOLE ARMENIAC). Hydragogue cathartic.

WARD'S ESSENCE FOR HEADACHE: Devised by Joshua Ward, it was later made official as Compound Liniment of CAMPHOR.

WARD'S LIQUID SWEAT: Devised by Joshua Ward, it was a tincture of OPIUM, CROCUS, CINNAMOMUM, and SAL TARTARI to be used as a diaphoretic.

WARD'S PASTE: Devised by Joshua Ward, it was a pile and

fistula-in-ano remedy later made official as Confection of PIPER NIGRUM.

WARD'S PILLS: Devised by Joshua Ward, it was a mixture of ANTIMONIUM VITRIFICATUM and SANGUIS DRACONIS. [13]

WARM BATH: Water heated to 85°F, prescribed to stimulate paralyzed muscles. Also see HEAT.

WARNER'S GOUT CORDIAL: A proprietary tincture of RHEI and SENNA; weak cathartic. [29]

WARWICK, POWDER OF EARL OF: A cathartic panacea said to have been devised by Robert Dudley, Earl of Warwick, in the early 17th century; made of SCAMMONY, ANTIMONIUM TARTARISATUM, and CREAM OF TARTAR. [13]

WATER CALTROP: Water chestnut, *Trapa natans*. Demulcent; used in poultices.

WATERCRESS: See NASTURTIUM AQUATICUM.

WATER DOCK: See HYDROLAPATHUM.

WATER HEMLOCK: See CICUTA.

WATER LILY: See NYMPHAEA ALBA.

WATER PEPPER: See PERSICARIA.

WEAPON SALVE: Same as SYMPATHETIC OINTMENT OF PARACELSUS.

WEDEL'S LAUDANUM: See LAUDANUM, WEDEL'S.

WHEY: See LAC and SOUR WHEY.

WHITE ARSENIC: Arsenic trioxide; see ARSENIC, WHITE.

WHITE HELLEBORE: Same as VERATRUM ALBUM.

WHITE LEAD: Lead monoxide, PbO. Used in compounding ointments and plasters because of its cooling, drying, and astringent properties. [23]

WHITE OXIDE OF BISMUTH: Same as SUB-NITRAS BISMUTHI.

WHITE POPPY: See PAPAVER ALBUM.

WHITE PRECIPITATE: Mercury ammonium chloride, $HgNH_2Cl$; however, in French *precipité blanc* means CALOMEL. Astringent and sedative ointment for skin disease. [23]

WHITE VITRIOL: Same as ZINCUM VITRIOLATUM.

WHITE WAX: See CERA ALBA.

WHITE WOOD: Same as LIRIODENDRON TULIPIFERA.

WHITWORTH'S RED BOTTLE: A medicine devised by "Dr."

John Taylor, a farrier of Whitworth, Lancashire, in the late 18th century, it contained CAMPHOR, ORIGANUM, and BUGLOSSUM.

WHORTLEBERRY: See UVA URSI.

WILD CUCUMBER: See CUCUMIS AGRESTIS.

WILD POTATO: Same as MECHOACANNA.

WILD RHUBARB: Same as MECHOACANNA.

WILLOW: See SALIX.

WIND ROOT: So-called because of its carminative action; same as ACLEPIAS DECUMBENS. [23]

WINE: See VINUM.

WINE OF THE TURKS: Same as LAUDANUM, because most opium came from Ottoman–ruled areas.

WINKLER'S ELECTUARY: Complex mixture for phthisis [see ref. 40, p. 225]

WINTERANUS [CORTEX]: Winter's bark, *Drimys winteri*, discovered in South America in 1577 by Capt. William Winter, Sir Francis Drake's vice-admiral. Aromatic tonic and antiscorbutic. CANELLA was often substituted for it. [15]

WINTERBERRY: See PRINOS VERTICILLATUS.

WINTER CHERRIES: See ALKEKENGI.

WINTERGREEN: May be GAULTHERIA, KALMIA LATIFOLIA, or PYROLA.

WITCH-HAZEL: See HAMAMELIS VIRGINIANA.

WOLFSBANE: See ACONITUM.

WOOD ASH: Same as LIXIVA.

WOOD LICE: See MILLEPEDA.

WOODS, DECOCTION OF THE: Same as DECOCTUM GUAIACI COMPOSITUM.

WORMSEED: Usually SANTONICUM, but sometimes BOTRYS.

WORMWOOD: See ABSINTHUM and ABSINTHUM MARITIMUM.

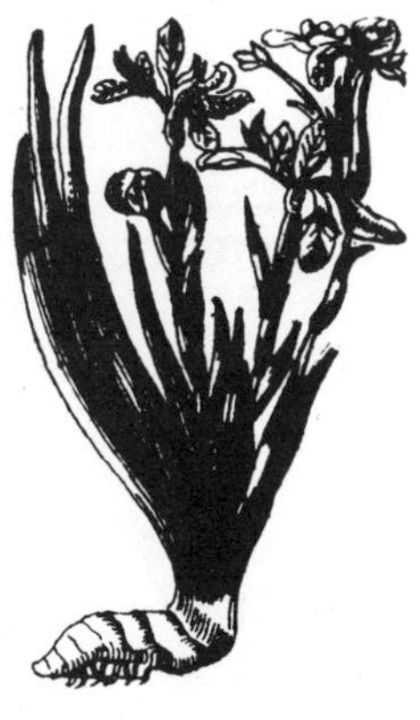

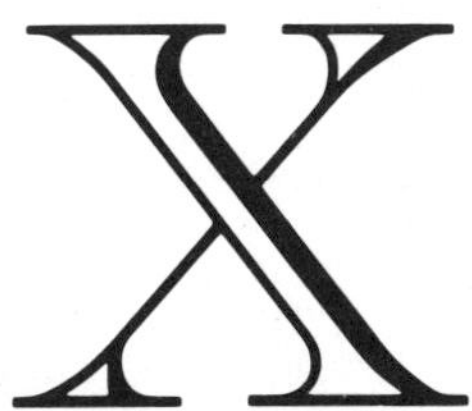

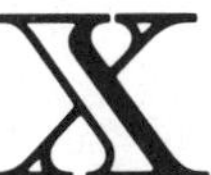

Xyris

XANTHORHIZA APIIFOLIA (or TINCTORIA): Stem and root of yellow root, *Xanthorhiza simplicissima*. A green dye with tonic bitter properties. [23,30]

XANTHOXYLUM [CLAVUS-HERCULIS]: Wood and root of prickly yellow wood, or yellow Hercules, *Zanthoxylum clava-Hercules*; see ARALIA SPINOSA. Narcotic, anodyne, antiepileptic, diaphoretic, and sialagogue; toothache remedy; discutient when applied topically. [23]

Xerocollyrium: A dry collyrium.

Xerophthalmica: Remedies for dry inflammations of the eyes.

XYRIS: See IRIS entries.

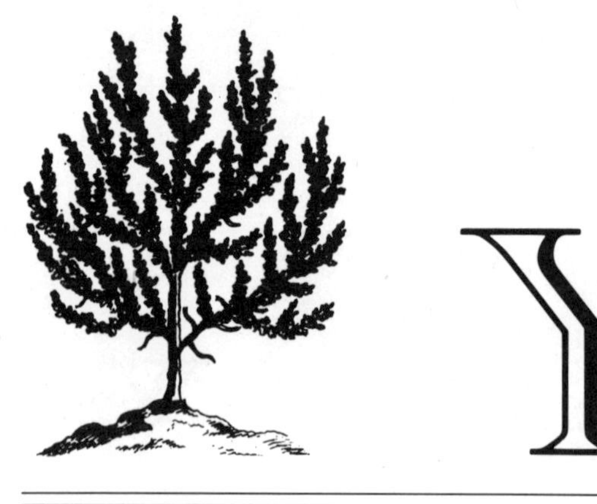

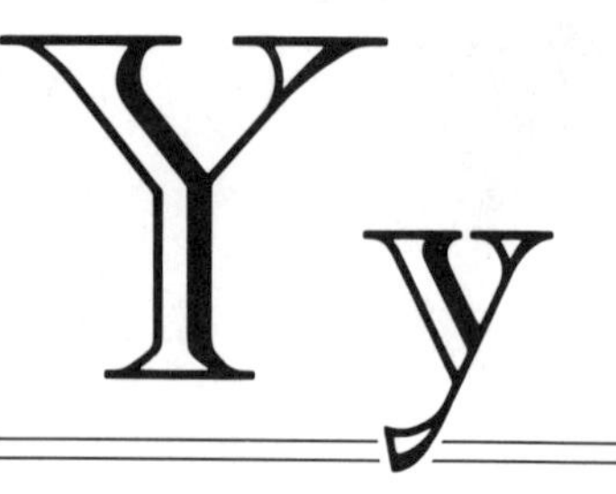

Yellow sandalwood

YELLOW BASILICON: Ointment made of CERA FLAVA, RESINA ALBA, OLIBANUM, and AXUNGUENTUM PORCINUM. Also see BASILICON OINTMENT.

YELLOW DOCK: Same as RUMEX CRISPUS.

YELLOW OINTMENT: Made with HYDRARGYRUS, SPIRIT OF NITER, and AXUNGUENTUM PORCINUM; prescribed for its mercurial effects. [15]

YELLOW ROOT: See XANTHORHIZA APIIFOLIA.

YELLOW SANDALWOOD: See SANTALUM CITRINUM.

YELLOW THISTLE: See ARGEMONE MEXICANA.

YELLOW WOOD: See XANTHOXYLUM.

YELLOW WAX: See CERA FLAVA.

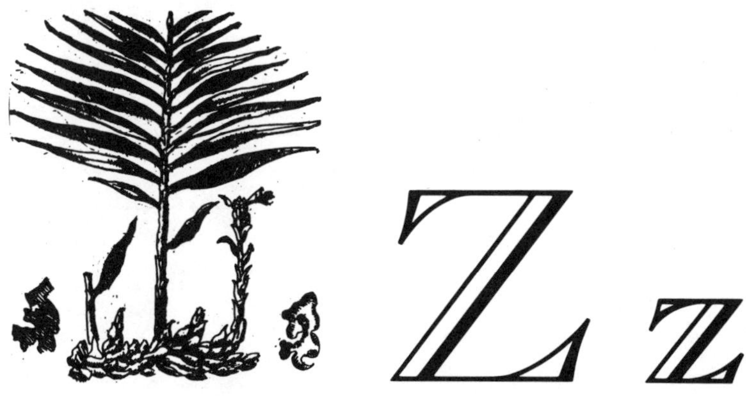

Zingiber

ZANTHOXYLUM: See ARALIA SPINOSA and XANTHOXYLUM.

ZEDOARIA: Root of zedoary, *Curcuma zedoaria*. Aromatic tonic. [15]

ZIBETHUM: Musky fluid from anal scent glands of African civet cat, *Viverra civetta*. Used chiefly in perfumes, rarely in medicines. [15]

ZINCI, BUTYRUM: "Butter of zinc," zinc chloride. Astringent. [15]

ZINCI CARBONAS: Same as CALAMINE.

ZINCI, FLORES: Same as ZINCUM USTUM.

ZINCUM PRAECIPITATUM: Zinc precipitated from ZINCUM VITRIOLATUM with VOLATILE ALKALI. Antispasmodic. [1]

ZINCUM USTUM: Zinc oxide. Tonic and antiepileptic; also used in collyria. [15,23]

ZINCUM VITRIOLATUM: Zinc sulfate. Used, rarely, as an antispasmodic and emetic; most often used externally as a styptic astringent. [1,15,23]

ZINGIBER: Root of ginger, *Zingiber officinale*. Used in tonics, to stimulate weak organs, and externally as a rubefacient. [23,29]

ZITTMAN'S DECOCTION: Introduced about 1750, it was made with CINNABAR and SARSAPARILLA. Escharotic and antisyphilitic.

ZIZYPHUS SPINA-CHRISTI: See JUJUBA.

APPENDIX

Protopharmacological Symbols

Although these symbols, which originated in alchemical usage, were seldom used by 18th-century physicians or apothecaries, their occurrence in the earlier medical literature warrants their inclusion here. The explanations of the symbols also explain, for instance, how Jupiter or Jove came to be associated with compounds of tin, Luna (the Moon) with silver, Mars with iron, Mercury with quicksilver, Saturn with lead, and Venus with copper. However, some explanations must be taken with a grain of salt; for instance, it cannot be confirmed that the ancient Romans considered Lithargyrus and Minium to be among the sons of the god Saturn, even if all three words are applied to lead salts.

The following pages are taken from John Woodall, *The Surgions Mate, or Military and Domestique Surgery* (London: Nicholas Bourne, 1639), pp. 248-260, courtesy of the Boston Medical Library. The same material appeared on pp. 312-328 of the first edition of Woodall's book (1617); the 1639 edition incorporated three more later treatises, and was republished in two later editions (1653 and 1655). The 1617 edition, along with plates from the later editions, was also published in a 1978 fascimile edited by John Kirkup (Kingsmead Press, Bath, England).

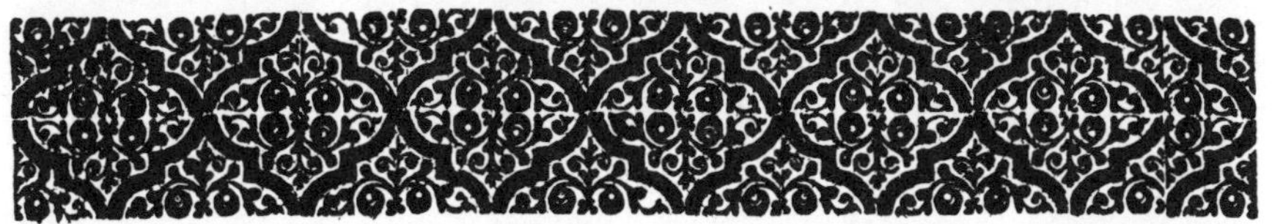

CHARACTERS AND THEIR INTERPRETATIONS.

And firſt of the ſeven Planets.

Saturnus. Plumbum ♄ · ♄ *Lead* Cold, deſiccative ſweet, diſcuſſing, mollificative, anodine, ſanative, laxative, mundificative, and yet full of deadly vapors.

Iupiter Stannum. ♃ · ♃ *Tin* Diaphoretick, laxative, deſiccative, ſanative, &c.

Mars Ferrum ♂ · ♂ *Iron, or Steele.* The greateſt ſhedder of bloud a ſure medicine for fluxes of bloud, and a great opener of obſtructions.

Sol. Aurum ☉ · ☉ *Gold* A great and ſure Cordiall, for it comforteth the heavy hearted, and is reputed the beſt medicine.

Venus. Cuperum ♀ · ♀ *Copper* Maketh ſundry needfull medicines for mans health, Phyſicall and Chirurgicall, viz: *Oleum, ſpiritus, & terra cum multis aliis.*

Mercurius. ☿ · ☿ *Quick-Silver* Is hot, cold, a friend, a foe, healing, killing, expelling, attracting, corroding, *& quid non?*

Luna. Argentum ☾ ☽ *Silver* A medicine never too often taken, a good reſtorative, a comfortable, and an anodine medicine, &c.

Other Characters Alphabetically.

Acetum. *Vineger of Beere* Good againſt inflammation, diſcuſſive, defenſative, comfortable, anodine, &c.

Acetum Vini. *Wine Vineger* A diſcuſſer, a cooler, a heater, a piercer, anodine, a conſumer, a cauſticke, and a veſicatory medicine, &c.

Acetum Diſtillatum. *Diſtil'd Vineger.* Is a vehicle that openeth minerall bodies and extracteth tinctures, &c.

Aer. *One of the 4 Elements* Without the which no creature ſubſiſteth.

Alumen *Allum Crude* Deſiccative, aſtringent, corroſive, mundificative ſanative, refrigerative, &c.

Alumen Combuſtum. *Allum Burnt* An eaſie and a good corroſive medicine, which alſo induceth a good cicatrix.

Alumen Plumoſum. *Allum Plume* A ſecret in reſtoring a withered member by a certaine hidden ſpecificall vertue it hath.

Albumen Ovorum. *Whites of Egges* Cold, defenſative, mollificative, healing, and good in reſtraining fluxes, &c.

Amalgama. A putting things together, or a terme of Art for putting together, viz: *fiat Almagama*, but more particularly it is meant of Mercury, with any other metall.

Antimonium. *Antimony* Vomitive, laxative, ſanative, diaphoretick, diaureticke, anodine, cauſticke, and full of deadly vapours, if it be not prevented, yet exceeding precious in healing, being diſcreetly uſed.

Antimonii

Antimonii Vitrum. *Glaſſe of Antimony or Stibiũ.* A forbidden medicine, and yet of Doctors uſed, and praiſe-worthy, if not abuſed.

Antimonii Regulus. *Antimony precipitate* This is but halfe a medicine, which afterward is uſed to be converted to Flores, Tincture, or ſome other good medicine.

Annus. *One yeare* From March the 25. till the return of the ſame.

Aqua. *Water* One of the foure elements of quality cold & moiſt.

Aqua Fortis. *Strong Water* Made by *Vulcans* Art of Coppras, Allome, and Salt-peeter, and diverſly other waies.

Aqua Regis. *A water to divide Gold.* This is made as the former, adding common ſalt, or rather *Sal Armoniacke.*

Aqua Vitæ. *Aquavita of Wine.* Aquavitæ diſtilled out of Wine is of excellent uſe for healing, and the chiefe cordiall in cheering the heart of man.

Arſenicum. *Arſnick* In taſte not unpleaſing, in triall deadly, yet a good outward healer many waies.

Auripigmentũ. *Orpiment* In taſte deadly, yet uſed of ſome inwardly for the cough, by fume with amber mixt, and outward in many medicines profitable.

Autumnus. *Harveſt* Or as it were an entrance to the Winter quarter.

Auriculum. *A chalke that containes gold.* Alſo gold calcined into powder being an entrance to *Aurum Potabile.*

Aurum Potabile. *Potable Gold* A Principall cordiall medicine, but very often adulterated, which being true, is precious.

Æſtas. *Sommer* This character is ſometimes uſed for Sommer and ſometimes for heate.

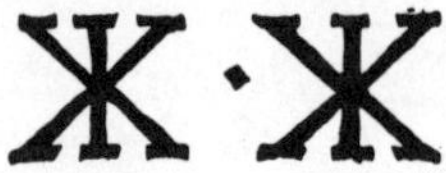

Æs. *Braſſe* This is but Copper mixed with *Lapis Calaminaris*, and prepared by *Vulcans* Art.

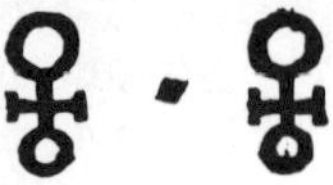

Balneum Mariæ. *Balnea Maria* Is an Artificiall diſtilling by a glaſſe Still ſet into a furnace in a Kettle of water, by the boyling of which, the ſubject contained in the glaſſe is diſtilled.

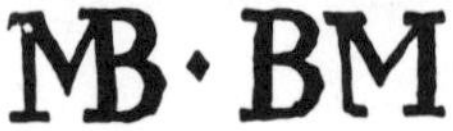

Bolus Armenus. *Fine bole* Is cordiall, deſiccative, reſtringent, ſanative, refrigerative, &c.

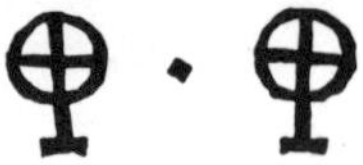

Bolus Communis. *Common Bole* Imitating the former, but farre weaker.

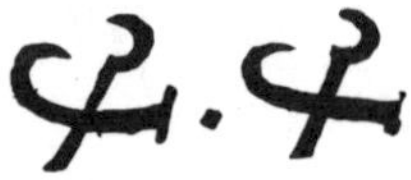

Borax Venetiæ. *Borax* This is a great opener of obſtructions of young women, and is excellent to lute glaſſes, and as a ſecond hand to Goldſmiths.

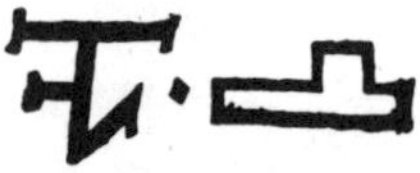

Calidus *Or rather Warme* Neither hot nor cold.

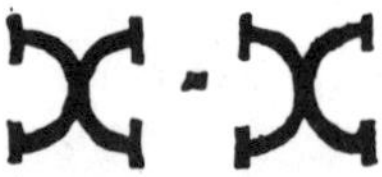

Calx. *Lime* Is abſterſive, deſiccative, cauſticke, ſanative.

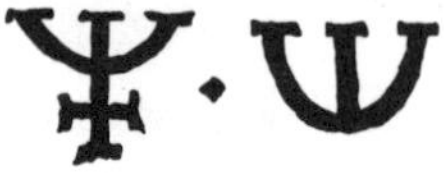

Calx Ovorum. *Lime of Eggeſhels* Is ſometime uſed in ſtrong reſtrictives, &c.

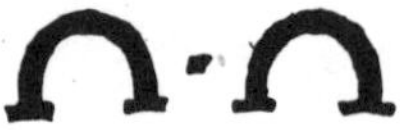

Calx Vive. *Unſlaked Lime* Chiefly uſed in Cauſticke medicines.

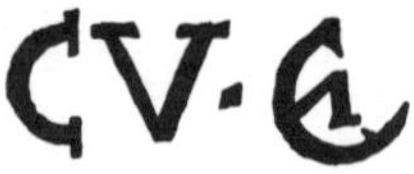

Chalybs. *Steele* The moſt valiant ſonne of *Mars*, it openeth obſtructions, and ſtayeth the fluxes, &c.

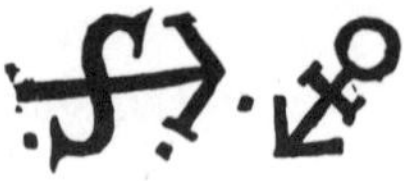

Calor. *Heate* This Character ſerveth not only for fire, but alſo for great heate.

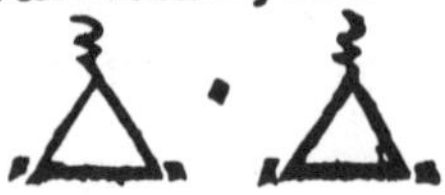

Calcinare.

Calcinare. *To Calcine.* Sometimes to burne to powder, and ſometimes to prepare by fire to a certaine height and colour.

Cementare *To Cement* Is by a mixture corroſive to adde to any metall pure, as Gold or ſilver, a higher tincture, and alſo to purifie the ſame yet further.

Ceruſſa Venetiæ. *Venice Ceruce* One of the off-ſpring of *Saturne*, ſanative, cooling, anodine, deſiccative, &c.

Cera. *Waxe* A bleſſed medicine outwards & inwards, of a temper neither exceedingly too hot, nor too cold, mollificative, ſanative, &c.

Cinnabrium. *Cinnabar* Found naturall and alſo compounded of Sulphur and Quick-ſilver, and uſed in Fumes, it ſpoyleth many, and healeth by chance ſome one in killing tenne.

Cineres Ligni. *Aſhes of Wood* Hereof are prepared many different medicines of value, in Phyſicke and Chirurgery, amongſt which the cauſticke ſtone, the ordinary Lixivium, &c.

Corallus Corallus Albus. *Corall white* Is Cordiall, cooling, drying, and beeing prepared Chymically, hath wonderfull vertues comfortative.

Corallus Rubeus. *Red Corall* This is as the former, but in vertues it farre exceedeth it. *Paracelſus* aſcribeth vertues infinite and wonderfull to red Corall, if it be perfectly red.

Colcothar. *Burnt Vitrioll, or Colcother.* A good cauſticke medicine, and alſo cooling, exſiccating, ſanative, mundificative, &c.

Crocus Martis. *Safron of Iron.* Good againſt *diſenterium*, *Gonorrea*, *Diarrhæa*, and generally all fluxes.

Crocus Veneris. *Safron of Copper* Or refined Verdigreaſe, as ſome affirme, but more truly is refined Æs Uſtum, it expelleth, drieth, mundifieth, & healeth.

Decoctio.

Decoctio.		*Boyling*	Is the boyling or decocting any medicine.
Digestio.		*Digesting*	Good digestion presageth good healing, but Chy-

micall digestion, *est gradus spagyricus similis ventriculo, per quem gradum materia coquitur melius ut puri ab impuro separatio fieri possit.*

Dies Et nox.		*Daie and Night*	Containing 24. houres.
Distillatio.		*Distilling*	Is the separation of the pure from the unpure,

performed by sublimation, and precipitation, but after many kindes and fashions.

Elementa.		*Not one of the foure Elements*	But a pure medicine made by Chymicall Art.

out of any good thing either Animall, vegetable, or minerall, *quere Labavii, lib. 2. Alchym. cap. 49.*

Filtrum.		*A felt*	This filtring with a felt, is a kinde of preparatiō of me-

dicines liquid, to purge them from their terrestriall parts.

Fimus Equinus.		*Horse-dung*	Chymists use to set their medicines in Horse-

dung to putrifie, and is an ancient and worthy worke rightly used. *Vicarius ejus est, BM. Balnia Maria.*

Fixatio.		*Fixing, or perfecting*	This is that all good Chymickes desire in their

workes, but few truely attaine it, but in stead of *fixatio*, they finde *vexatio satis, & ultimo mendicatum ire.*

Flos Æris.		*Verdigrease*	Called commonly *viride as*, and Verdigrease be-

ing the rust of Copper, it is a good astringent, disiccative, and corrosive medicament.

Gradus. G1 · G2 · G3 A degree first, second, or third, as you see them described with their severall figures.

Gummi. · *Gumme* · Of any kinde is so described, but the single Character is most used.

Hyems. · *Winter* This Character is also used for cold by some Writers.

Ignis. · *Fire* As well naturall as artificiall, actuall as potentiall, but the first is most in use.

Lapis Magnetis. · *The Loadstone* A jewel precious, for value far exceeding the Diamond, of the tribe of *Mars*, in qualitie attractive and sanative.

Lues Venerea. · *The venereall disease* This is a Catholike plague containing almost all diseases in one, being seldome perfectly healed.

Luna Crescens. · *The Moone increasing* Or the first and second quarter of the Moone.

Luna Decrescens. · *The Moone decreasing* Of the two last quarters of the Moone.

Lapis Prunella. · *A stone made of Salniter* This is good against toothache and inflammations, and for sores of the mouth and throat, and also against hot fevers inwardly taken.

Lapis Calaminaris. · *Calamint Stone* Is a stone which changeth Copper into Brasse, it is desiccative, and excelleth in Lotions for the eyes, &c.

Lapis Hematites. *Bloud-stone* This stone is used to stench bleeding inwardly and outwardly, and hath many other vertues medicinable.

Lapis Sabuloſus. This is a great ſecret n curing a fracture being daily given the partie, ℥j. and alſo mixed with the outward medicine, and applyed to the griefe.

Lapis Granatus. *The Granat Stone* This is a Jewell precious in medicine, but not commonly uſed.

Lateres. *Stones* Or Brickes for farnaſis or otherwaies.

Lateres Cribrati. *Powder of Brickes* It is often uſed in preparing medicines as well to make good Lute, as alſo for divers other needfull uſes.

Loxivium or Lixivium. *Lye made of aſhes* This is many waies uſed very profitable in healing outwardly and inwardly, and for cauſtick medicines it is the beſt.

Limatura Martis. *Filings of Iron* Uſed for the making of *Crocus Martis*.

Lutum Sapientia *Lute uſed of the Philoſophers* Is an artificiall mixture of Clay; for the making of furnaſes, and luting glaſſes and pots for diſtillation.

Lutum Commune. *Lute Common* Made of good clay, with the flox of wooll, and ſalt commonly, but there is as many ſeveral Lutes that Chymiſts do know

Lythargirus Auri. *Litharge of Gold* One of the ſons of *Saturne*, and is partly ſo tearmed, for that the teſts which refine Gold through Lead, after are made into Litharge, I meane the *Saturne* into them.

Lythargirus Argenti. *Litharge of Silver* One of the ſons of *Saturne*, ſuppoſed to proceed of *Luna* as aforeſaid, but indeed this and the firſt are ſent daily from *Holland*, made onely of Lead.

Lythargirus Plumbi. *Litharge of Lead* One other of the ſonnes of *Saturne*, and is made by every Plumber out of that part of *Saturne* which waſteth to a hardneſſe in melting.

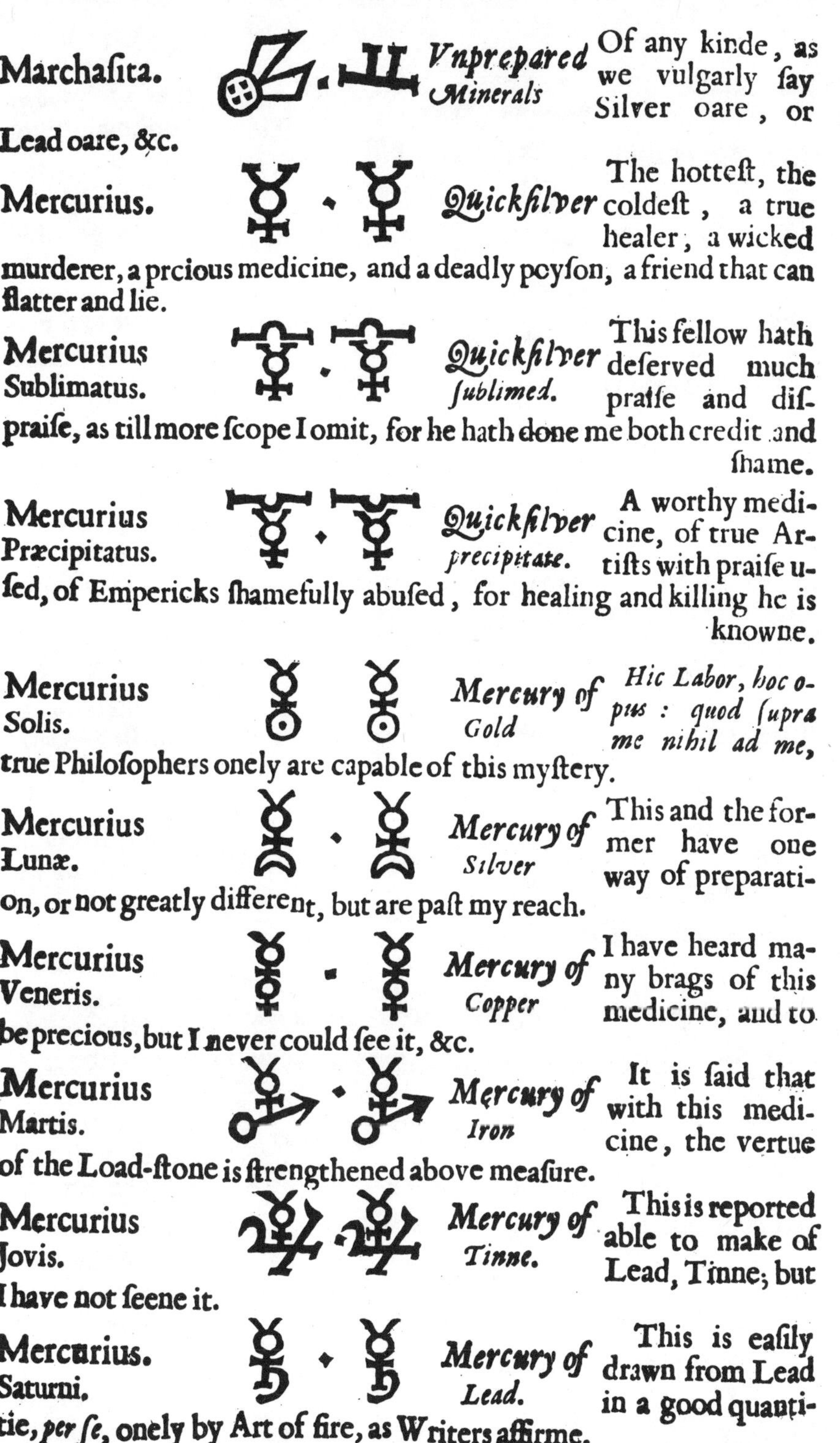

Marchasita. *Unprepared Minerals* Of any kinde, as we vulgarly say Silver oare, or Lead oare, &c.

Mercurius. *Quickſilver* The hotteſt, the coldeſt, a true healer, a wicked murderer, a prcious medicine, and a deadly poyſon, a friend that can flatter and lie.

Mercurius Sublimatus. *Quickſilver ſublimed.* This fellow hath deſerved much praiſe and diſpraiſe, as till more ſcope I omit, for he hath done me both credit and ſhame.

Mercurius Præcipitatus. *Quickſilver precipitate.* A worthy medicine, of true Artiſts with praiſe uſed, of Empericks ſhamefully abuſed, for healing and killing he is knowne.

Mercurius Solis. *Mercury of Gold* *Hic Labor, hoc opus: quod ſupra me nihil ad me,* true Philoſophers onely are capable of this myſtery.

Mercurius Lunæ. *Mercury of Silver* This and the former have one way of preparation, or not greatly different, but are paſt my reach.

Mercurius Veneris. *Mercury of Copper* I have heard many brags of this medicine, and to be precious, but I never could ſee it, &c.

Mercurius Martis. *Mercury of Iron* It is ſaid that with this medicine, the vertue of the Load-ſtone is ſtrengthened above meaſure.

Mercurius Jovis. *Mercury of Tinne.* This is reported able to make of Lead, Tinne; but I have not ſeene it.

Mercurius. Saturni. *Mercury of Lead.* This is eaſily drawn from Lead in a good quantitie, *per ſe*, onely by Art of fire, as Writers affirme.

Menſis. *One moneth* Containing 28. daies, and 28. nights, or foure whole weekes.

Minium. Or red Lead — Is one of the ſons of *Saturne*, cooling, drying, repelling, healing, mollifying, diſcuſſing, &c.

Minutum. *One Minute* — The ſixtieth part of one houre.

Mel. M·M *Honey* — Honey is Laxative, mundificative, mollificative, ſanative, &c.

Oleum. *Oyle of any kinde* — And ſometimes taken for Sulphur, is as if you would ſay, take from *Guaiacum* his *Sal*, *Sulphur*, and *Mercury*, by his Sulphur you muſt underſtand his oyly part, &c.

Phlegma. *A Plegma* — It is uſed for any diſtilled water which is void of Spirit, as Roſe water.

Piger Henricus. *Slow Hemick* — An inſtrument for diſtilling, ſo called, for his exceeding ſlowneſſe.

Plumbum Philoſophorum. *Philoſophers Lead* — This preparation is myſticall, and above my reach, the ſame Character is alſo uſed for the Philoſophers ſtone.

Pulvis. *Powder of any thing* — Any fine powder, and ſometimes it is taken for ſubtill flores, and fine ſpirits of any medicine.

Purificare. *To Purifie* — Either by ſublimation, or by precipitation, or any kinde of purifying or cleanſing.

Putrefactio. *Putrifie* — Is diſſolving or opening of mixed Minerals bodies by a naturall, warme, and moiſt putrefaction, namely, by *fimus equinus, vel ejus Vicarius, MB.*

Quinta Eſſentia.	QE · QE	*Quinta Eſſentia*	A permament Eſſentiall well digeſted medicine,

without groſſe ſuperfluities, drawne from any ſubſtance either Animall, Vegetable, or Minerall.

Quinta Eſſentia vini.	· QEV	*The Quinteſſence of Wine*	This is alſo called *Aquavitæ*, and *Aqua*

Cœleſtis, and *Alcole vini*, and *Aqua Ardens*, with many other names.

Realgar.		*A kinde of Ratsbane*	A thing ſeldome uſed in healing, though ſome-

times uſed in Alchymy.

Reverberatio.			A preparation Chymicall by fire.
Retorta.		*A retort of Glaſſe*	

Sublimare.		*To ſublime*	Or to cauſe to aſcend by fire or Art of diſtilling

very many waies.

Sulphur.		*Brimſtone*	Diſcuſſive, ſanative, deſiccative, anodine, repercuſſive, &c.
Sulphur Philoſophorum.		*Perfect Sulphur vix cognitum*	A true eſſentiall, perfect, and univer-

ſall medicament out of *Sol*.

Sal Communis.		*Common Salt*	Diſcuſſive, mundificative, ſanative, and moſt preci-

ous for the life of man.

Sal Gemmæ.		*Precious ſalt like Chryſtall*	A Chryſtaline Salt, naturally growing in mines

in Polonia, neere the Citie of Cracovia, &c.

Sal Petræ.		*Salt Peeter*	A Salt of a wonderfull kinde and breeding, with ef-

fects admirable both good and evill.

Sal Amoniacum. — *Salt Amoniack* — Growes naturally in Turky, but is commonly made of *Sal Alkali*, common Salt, Urin, &c. *Teste Andrea libavio.*

Sal Alkali. — *A Salt of an heard called Kali* — A kinde of vegetable Salt, but *Paracelsus* termeth every vegetable Salt *Alkaly*.

Sal Colcotharis. — *A salt out of Deadhead* — A Salt drawne from the *Caput mortuum*, and commonly called Deadhead, which is exceeding astringent and drying.

Sal Tartari. — *A Salt of Argall* — The Salt of Tartar or wine Lees a medicine of many great vertues, both of it selfe, and also for making other medicines.

Succinum Album. — *White Amber* — Commeth from Prutia & is a Cordiall medicine, diaureticke, diaphoreticke, laxative, and generally opening all obstructions.

Succinum Citrinum. — *Yellow Amber* — Like the former, but not so good, yet from this is an excellent oyle drawne, serving for many especiall medicines inward and outward.

Spiritus Vini. — *Spirit of Wine* — A pure and essentiall substance, cordiall, and of infinite other vertues, Liquid, yet wholy combustible.

Sapo. — *Sope* — A good medicine attractive, mollificative, &c.

Stratum Super Stratum. — *Two medicines laid one upon another* — A terme of Art often used, viz: *fiat stratum, super stratum*, that is, first put in of the one, and then of the other till all be in.

Solutio. — *Opening* — The opening of minerall bodies diversly by *Vulcans* Art.

Sigillum Hermetis. — *Hermes his Seale* — A kinde of Luting or sealing of Glasses by a more excellent manner.

Terra.	*Earth*	Commonly taken for potters earth to make Lute of.
Tigillum.	*A melting pot*	A pot wherewith Gold-ſmiths and other Artiſts uſe to melt metals or medicines in, called alſo a Crucible.
Talcum.	*Talke*	This minerall is ſcarce well known yet, the oyle therof is much extolled for beautifying the skinne.
Tutia.	*Tutty*	A medicine commonly knowne, and is made of the ſcum of Copper, or of Copper by combuſtion.
Tartarus.	*Argall*	Is the Lees of wine dried, which makes many profitable medicines, artificially prepared.
Tumores.	*Tumors*	And alſo any Apoſtum or ſwelling, whereſoever in mans body.
Turbith Minerall.	*Turbith Minerall*	This with ſome additaments artificiall, well prepared, is precious in the cure of the French pox.

Vlcus.	*An Vlcer*	This is the ancient Character for an Ulcer, & ſome Authors, have uſed the ſame for a wound.
Vitriolum.	*Coppras*	It is beſt which is made of Copper.
Vitrum.	*Glaſſe*	It is uſed for a Glaſſe Still, and alſo for any other kinde of glaſſe.
Vrina.	*Vrine*	Mans urine or childrens urine, it is commonly uſed in Alchymie, and ſome uſe it in fomentations, and otherwiſe in Chirurgery and Phyſicke.